A COMPREHENSIVE

HEALTH
AND
WEALTH
MANAGEMENT

for a worry-free retirement!

Dear Ender and Carmen,
Wishing you good health, happiness,
and prosperity.

JAMES M. LUONGO, CLU, CHFC

A Comprehensive Guide to Health and Wealth Management for a Worry-Free Retirement

Copyright © 2020 by James M. Luongo

All rights reserved. No part of this publication may be reproduced, distributed, or transmitted in any form or by any means, including photocopying, recording, or other electronic or mechanical methods, without the prior written permission of the publisher or author, except in the case of brief quotations embodied in critical reviews and certain other noncommercial uses permitted by copyright law. For permission requests or to contact the author, visit: https://www.luongowealthmanagement.com/.

ISBN-10: 8-686-89937-7
ISBN-13: 979-8-686-89937-7

Printed in the United States of America

The content of this book is for general informational purposes only. It is not meant to be used, nor should it be used, to diagnose or treat any medical condition or to replace the services of your physician or other healthcare provider. The advice and strategies contained in the book may not be suitable for all readers. Please consult your healthcare provider for any questions that you may have about your own medical situation. Neither the author, publisher, IIN, LPL Financial, nor any of their employees or representatives, guarantees the accuracy of information in this book or its usefulness to a particular reader, nor are they responsible for any damage or negative consequence that may result from any treatment, action taken, or inaction, by any person reading or following the information in this book.

This information is not intended to be a substitute for specific individualized tax or legal advice. We suggest that you discuss your specific situation with a qualified tax or legal advisor. Stock market CDs pose inherent risks, such as market and liquidity risks. Returns are not guaranteed, and principal is only guaranteed when held to maturity. If purchasers sell their CDs prior to maturity, they may receive more or less than their original investment. Past performance of any indices is not a predictor of future results. CD returns may not track full performance of the indices themselves. May not be suitable for all investors. Investors should carefully read the related term sheet and prospectus and/or disclosure statement before investing. Structured product CDs may be treated differently than traditional CDs for tax purposes and investors should consult their tax advisors. Investing in mutual funds involves risk, including possible loss of principal. Stock investing involves risk, including loss of principal. Fixed and variable annuities are suitable for long-term investing, such as retirement investing. Gains from tax-deferred investments are taxable as ordinary income upon withdrawal. Guarantees are based on the claims paying ability of the issuing company. Withdrawals made prior to age 59 ½ are subject to a 10% IRS penalty tax and surrender charges may apply. Variable annuities are subject to market risk and may lose value. Riders are additional guarantee options that are available to an annuity or life insurance contract holder. While some riders are part of an existing contract, many others may carry additional fees, charges and restrictions, and the policy holder should review their contract carefully before purchasing. Guarantees are based on the claims paying ability of the issuing insurance company.

I dedicate this book to my wife, Gail,
and my children, Michael and Amanda,
for their encouragement and support during the
countless hours that I spent writing this book.
I also dedicate this book to my parents,
my brothers, and my extended family.

CONTENTS:

Acknowledgments	7
Forward	9
Introduction	11

Part I: Health Management — 17

Introduction		19
Chapter 1:	Making America Healthy	21
Chapter 2:	My Transformation	25
Chapter 3:	Air Out Your Home and Your Office	37
Chapter 4:	Reduce Exposure to Toxins	39
Chapter 5:	Get Some Sunlight	47
Chapter 6:	Manage Stress and Anxiety	49
Chapter 7:	Get Sufficient Sleep and Rest	55
Chapter 8:	Get Up and Exercise	59
Chapter 9:	Drink Plenty of Water	65
Chapter 10:	Balance Your Gut Bacteria to Improve Your Health and Immunity	69
Chapter 11:	Improve Your Diet	73
Chapter 12:	Take Charge of Your Healthcare Decisions	119
Chapter 13:	Cancer	125
Chapter 14:	Maintain a Routine	131
Chapter 15:	Balance Your Life	133
Chapter 16:	Fixing Our Healthcare Crisis	135
Summary		137
Recommended Sources for Health Management		139

Part II: Wealth Management — 141

Introduction — 143

Chapter 1: Healthcare Spending Risk — 147

Chapter 2: Long-Term Care Risk — 155

Chapter 3: The Death or Divorce of a Spouse/Partner — 161

Chapter 4: Not Having a Proper Estate Plan — 177

Chapter 5: Taxes in Retirement — 183

Chapter 6: Bad Advice, Scams, Fraud, and Identity Theft — 201

Chapter 7: Longevity Risk — 209

Chapter 8: Withdrawal Risk — 219

Chapter 9: Sequence of Return Risk — 221

Chapter 10: Investment Risk — 227

Chapter 11: Investment Behavior — 235

Chapter 12: Financial Risk Management Strategies — 239

Summary — 257

References — 259

ACKNOWLEDGMENTS

A special thanks to Cathy Pisaturo and A. Barbara Owen for editing the book and to Amie Olson for the interior and book cover design.

FORWARD

This book was inspired by my experiences working in the financial services industry for over thirty years, as well as my experience at the Institute for Integrative Nutrition® (IIN), where I received training in holistic wellness and health coaching. I feel very fortunate to work as a financial advisor, in a field that I truly enjoy, and to work with so many wonderful people. I am also very fortunate to enjoy good health and a balanced life.

This book combines a detailed discussion about health and wealth management. Building wealth and enjoying good health takes patience, hard work, and discipline, and must be balanced with other facets of your life. Just as a person cannot expect to wake up one day and suddenly become wealthy, they should not expect to enjoy good health without putting in some effort and dedication towards being healthy. The good news is that, even if you have a late start, you can still build a healthier you. To truly enjoy retirement, it is imperative to develop healthy habits and maintain good health, and to have a solid retirement plan in place so you can pursue your interests and hobbies, and spend time with family and friends, without worrying about running out of money. This book can help in both areas. Enjoy it in good health and wealth!

INTRODUCTION

"All parts of the body which have a function, if used in moderation and exercised in labors in which each is accustomed, become thereby healthy, well developed and age more slowly, but if unused they become liable to disease, defective in growth, and age quickly."

~ Hippocrates

Two Brothers, Jack and Bill meet for lunch.

Jack is 67 years old and in great physical shape. He exercises daily, follows a healthy diet, doesn't drink or smoke, sleeps 7-8 hours every night, and enjoys a low-stress lifestyle. He has worked for 45 years and, even though he has not saved as much as he would have liked, he is hoping to retire soon and travel with his wife, as they have always dreamed. He doesn't have a pension, so the only source of guaranteed income that he and his wife will have in retirement is Social Security. Jack turns to Bill, and says, "I went to a financial advisor the other day and completed a retirement analysis. I was hoping he would tell me that I can finally retire. Instead, he told me I would have to work for another ten years, or we would most likely outlive our money. We were so disappointed, since we were hoping to travel and spend a lot of time with our grandchildren. But you know what the worst part was? He had the nerve to say to me, 'At least you have your health!'"

Bill is 65 years old, very wealthy, and recently retired. He had diligently planned for his retirement, saving and investing at an early age. He had worked very hard to build a successful business, which he recently sold for $10,000,000. He doesn't have any financial concerns and was looking forward to his retirement years. Unfortunately, his long hours and hard work have taken a toll on his health, because he didn't exercise, he ate a lot of unhealthy foods, he drank too much, and he was constantly overstressed, and sleep deprived. He is overweight, suffers from diabetes, has a heart condition, and has chronic knee pain from carrying excess weight for 30 years. He takes six different medications to "manage" his health. Though he, too, was hoping to travel during his retirement, the only traveling he does is going back and forth to doctors' offices. Bill turns to Jack and says, "Oh yeah, I went to see my cardiologist today, and she gave me some terrible news. I have congestive heart failure, and it's only going to get worse over time. You know what she had the nerve to say? 'At least you have your wealth!'"

So, what's the point of this story? The point is, to truly enjoy a long and active retirement, you need to have a plan for *both* health and wealth management. What good is one without the other? As a financial advisor, I have met many people who are financially successful, but are in poor health. They worked hard, carefully saved and invested for their financial future. Yes, this meticulous planning has enabled them to accumulate enough money to enjoy their retirement years. However, they neglected to take care of their health so, over time, they have developed degenerative diseases that require ongoing treatment. Now, much of their free time in retirement is spent in doctors' offices or in hospitals; they are not traveling and spending time with their family and friends, as they had envisioned.

Accumulating wealth takes patience, hard work, and discipline; it doesn't happen by chance. I think most people realize this. You don't just wake up one day and suddenly find that you're wealthy. The same is true about good health. You don't just wake up one day to find yourself fit and healthy. Good health and wellness also takes patience, hard work, and discipline. As with accumulating wealth, the sooner you start your path towards good health, the better.

Humans are complex organisms. Our bodies were intended to eat whole, natural foods, not processed ones. By design, our bodies were meant to move often, not to sit for most of the day. We were meant to spend time outdoors, in the sun and fresh air, not indoors under artificial light, and amid stale, recycled air. We need to respect and take good care of our own body, the way we would want someone else to treat it if they could borrow it for a day.

Most organisms on our planet eat a diet of natural foods. But many humans eat a diet of processed foods and suffer from degenerative diseases. Even our pets, who eat the processed foods that we feed them, are experiencing the same degenerative diseases from which we suffer. "Today there are simply too many sick people. Nature didn't create a situation where so many human beings are doomed to suffer from all kinds of major ailments such as cancer, and to die in a slowly deteriorating often agonizingly painful process, or linger on for years before death often thankfully comes. This condition was created by man."[1]

Although the focus of this book is geared toward retirees and pre-retirees, the first section on health management is applicable to all age groups. It is never too early to develop good health habits, and it is never too late to improve your less-than-stellar health.

Before I made significant changes in my own life, I was headed in the same health direction as that of a typical person who does not pay much attention to what he eats.

Age and Changes in Health

20s

Many people in their 20s are finishing school or starting careers. If you have not already started at this point, this is the time to start paying attention to your health. When I started college, I weighed 155 pounds. I was active and played soccer in my freshman and sophomore years. But four years of eating the wrong foods, drinking too much alcohol, and (but for a couple of seasons of soccer) leading a mostly sedentary life, led to a weight gain of about 13 pounds. When I graduated college in 1988, I weighed about 168 pounds, which, for my 5'7" frame, wasn't terrible, but wasn't great either. Not much has changed for today's youth. Young people are still consuming way too many unhealthy foods, and too much alcohol. During your 20s, if you don't start to eat a better diet - including the elimination of fried foods - and don't have a consistent exercise regimen, you will begin to put on weight, as I did, because you simply cannot get away with the same lifestyle that you were able to get away with as a teenager. Today, many teenagers and pre-teens are overweight due to a poor diet and lack of exercise, suggesting attention to health really needs to start at an even earlier age.

30s

When you reach your 30s, you might be married and starting a family. This is when your diet and exercise routine might suffer even more. Exhaustion and a busy schedule leave no time to cook healthy meals (which typically take longer to prepare), or to exercise. You try to get by on less sleep, while your advancing career and family responsibilities increase your stress levels. You notice that you are putting on additional weight and have less energy. When you go for your annual physical, your doctor tells you that your lab results don't look good, and you need to lose weight and start exercising. Your doctor might even suggest medications for your pre-hypertension, pre-diabetes, or increasing cholesterol numbers. This was the time in my life when I started putting on even more weight, and really getting out of shape.

40s

At this point in life, you might be climbing the corporate ladder and working too many hours. You sleep less, wake up exhausted, and cannot start the day without two cups of coffee or other caffeinated drinks. A typical diet consists of way too much sugar and carbohydrates. You have even less energy, and you are barely getting through the day. You now have hypertension and high cholesterol, and you are taking several prescription medications to manage your symptoms. You become anxious and depressed, and your doctor prescribes anti-anxiety and antidepressant meds. Life seems overwhelming at this point. When I reached my early to mid-40s, I was in the worst shape of my life. Fortunately (perhaps miraculously), I did not need any medications at that time, but I undoubtedly was headed in that direction. This is also the time in my life when my brother became seriously ill, prompting me to begin the transformation to where I am today.

50s

At this point in your life, you gain even more weight, and you are now diabetic. In addition to the numerous prescription drugs you are taking, you are also giving yourself daily insulin injections. You start hearing about friends from high school or college dying suddenly of a heart attack or being diagnosed with cancer. This makes you even more anxious. You start to realize that you have to do something differently, or you will be headed down the same path as your friends. So, you cut down on your junk food, you start to exercise, you try to get more sleep, but things don't improve much. You think, maybe it's too late, the damage is already done, maybe it's all hereditary anyway, so what's the use, and you give up.

60s

You look forward to retirement and enjoying the "good life," but you are now in very poor health. You are in constant pain, suffer from anxiety, and cannot sleep. You suffer a heart attack and need quadruple bypass surgery. You survive, but you are now taking many additional medications to manage your symptoms, and you feel lousy all the time.

70s and 80s (if you make it that long)

You are now retired. You had hoped to travel, but the only traveling you do is back and forth to doctors' offices and hospitals. You now start to show signs of dementia. You find blood in your stool and go for a colonoscopy to find out that you have colon cancer. Your doctor tells you that you will need surgery, radiation, and chemotherapy, and that there is a good chance you will have to wear a colostomy bag for the remainder of your life.

This is quite a depressing scenario, and not one that anyone hopes for. Unfortunately, this rings true for far too many people. But it does not have to be this way. In fact, even if things have gotten this bad for you, or close to it, many degenerative diseases that take years to develop are still reversible.

Once you gain control of your health, your symptoms can slowly start to dissipate, and your body can start to heal. Over time, you will start to feel better, and with the approval of your doctor, you may get off some, if not all, of your medications. You can then, finally, start to live the life you deserve, and enjoy the wealth you have accumulated.

Every decision in life, whether good or bad, will affect the outcome of both your health and your wealth. Saving money and living below your means when you are young, eating well, exercising regularly, getting enough sleep and rest, managing stress, and reducing exposure to toxins - all will pay dividends in the future. See how easy it is to tie in health and wealth management together?

Depending on your age, you may have plenty of time or little time to get your health and your finances in order before you retire. This book can help in both aspects.

How do you envision your retirement?

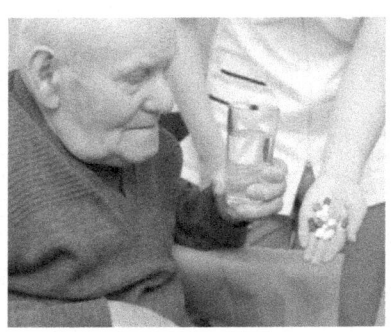
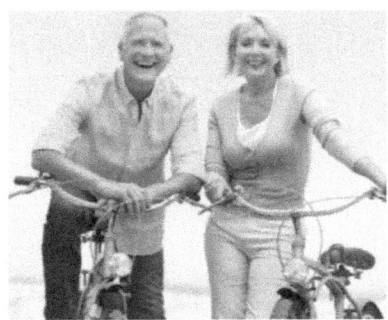

This book is divided into two sections. Part I focuses on health management because without good health, no amount of wealth is meaningful. Part II's focus on wealth management helps you prepare for retirement, discusses financial risks in retirement, and suggests some strategies to help mitigate these risks. As I said earlier, I wrote this book with the pre-retiree and retiree in mind, but many of the concepts in this book, particularly in Part I, are applicable to people of all ages.

PART I: HEALTH MANAGEMENT

INTRODUCTION

In this section, I will discuss how I vastly improved my health and became passionate about health management. I will suggest ways to improve your health through diet, exercise, stress reduction, sleep and relaxation, detoxification/elimination, and will address other components of your life that affect your health. Let's get started.

CHAPTER 1:
MAKING AMERICA HEALTHY

"A wise man should consider that health is the greatest of human blessings, and learn by his own thought to derive benefit from his illnesses."

~ Hippocrates

Imagine a world where there are no degenerative diseases. This means no cancer, no heart disease, no diabetes, and no autoimmune diseases, period! People would have normal blood sugar levels, normal blood pressures, and normal cholesterol levels. There would be no more obesity, no more arthritis, and no needless suffering. People would not have to take handfuls of pills each day. Wouldn't this be a fantastic world? Yes, but the world I describe is pure fantasy. If fewer and fewer people were taking expensive drugs, pharmaceutical companies would go out of business. Doctors and hospitals would have very few sick patients to treat, and they, too, would struggle to stay in business. Food manufacturers would have to produce healthier foods to remain in business. Since drug companies, doctors, and hospitals make a lot of money when people get sick, there is hardly any incentive for change.

Drug companies don't want to cure people, they just want to manage the symptoms of disease. They hope that people start taking their drugs at an early age and continue taking them for life. Drug companies are extremely profitable and continue to create new and better drugs to "cure" our every ill. But drugs don't cure underlying diseases, they only treat the symptoms. They are a quick fix, a band aid. People don't come down with a degenerative disease because of a lack of drugs in their body.

While I believe that most doctors genuinely care about helping their patients, many are trained to diagnose and treat patients with drugs. They receive very little training and education on diet; some doctors don't even believe that diet plays a role in their patients' overall health. In addition, their very busy schedules allow them to spend only 5-10 minutes per patient, as they need to see many patients to maintain a profitable practice. Hospitals are fantastic at treating patients that have suffered from accidents, heart attacks, and other acute conditions. But when it comes to treating degenerative diseases, hospitals are terrible, especially with respect to the food that they provide to patients.

Food manufacturers will continue to produce processed "food" products, which can sit on store shelves for long periods of time. The longevity of these products increases the manufacturers' profits.

So, in the end, it turns out that it is not in anyone else's best interest but your own to change the status-quo. For drug companies, doctors, hospitals, and the food industry, it all boils down to profits. If those industries were to put our interests ahead of their own, we would be a much healthier nation.

Life expectancies have risen greatly over time. According to the National Center for Health Statistics, in 1950, the average life expectancy of an American born that year was 68.2 years, while the average life expectancy of an American born in 2017 is 78.6 years.[1] But, as a nation, our health has declined dramatically. In the 1950s, only about 10% of U.S. adults were classified as obese. In 2011-2012, approximately 35% of U.S. adults were obese - an increase of 3½ times.[2] Currently, 66% of American adults are overweight or obese, and nearly 30% of children are overweight or obese.[3] That's a huge number, and a big increase in only 8 years!

Good health practices encompass the whole body, including the physiological side and the psychological side. This includes nutrition obtained from whole foods, drinking adequate amounts of water, consistent elimination of body wastes and toxins, sufficient exercise, adequate sleep and rest, modest to low stress, and a positive attitude towards life. According to Art Waerland, Ph.D., the originator of a system of health restoration that was the basis for establishing many health clinics in Europe, "By means of the blood and nervous system, all the different organs and minutest parts of the body are bound together in an exquisitely adjusted homogeneous cell community, in which normally, everything functions in normal harmony. A disturbance in any one part affects the whole."[4]

So, what if you're motivated to lose weight, improve your health, reduce your dependency on prescription drugs, sleep better, have more energy, and not walk around in a constant fog? What should you do? I believe the answer is to start taking your health very seriously (even if you don't currently have any present health problems), and to make it a top priority. Take the time to educate yourself on health and nutrition. Read articles and books on the subject, search the internet for accurate and truthful information, watch documentaries on food and health (there are many on Netflix and YouTube), shop at health food stores, learn to read and understand the ingredients of every food product before you buy it, and be very particular about where you dine out. About 8-9 years ago, this is exactly what I did. Not only did I lose weight - which I have managed to keep off - but I improved my health, my energy, and my outlook on life, and I made health and wellness a passion of mine.

CHAPTER 2:
MY TRANSFORMATION

"If we could give every individual the right amount of nourishment and exercise, not too little and not too much, we would have found the safest way to health."

~ Hippocrates

I was not always as fit and healthy as I am today at the age of 53. Here are some pictures of me when I was in my 30s and 40s.

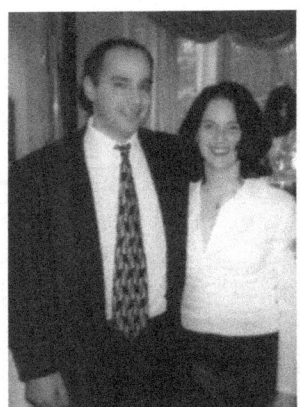 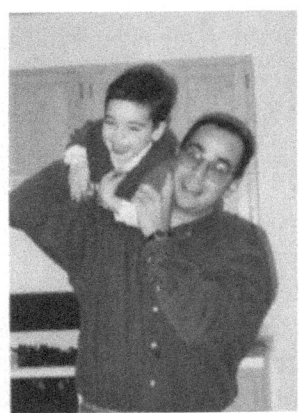 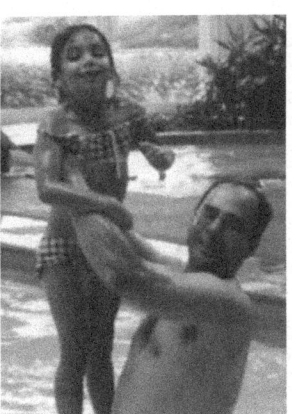

Here is a picture taken of me in 2019 at the age of 52.

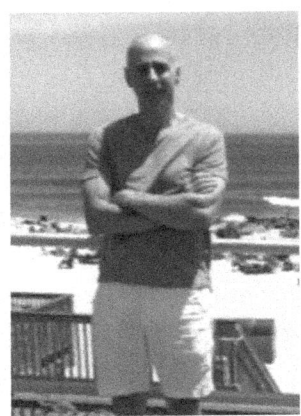

Recently, while flying to California on a business trip, I had a chance to reflect on my personal journey to health and wellness. Let me explain how I became so passionate about the subject. Throughout my life, I have always been relatively active playing sports and working out. Still, in my 20s and 30s, I began to put on weight, and found that no matter how hard I worked out, I just could not lose weight. I was convinced, then, that gaining weight was a natural aging process, and I proceeded to put on more weight. My weight peaked in my mid-40s when I reached 180 pounds (about 35 pounds more than I weigh today). This was a lot of weight for my 5'7" frame. I did not think of myself as fat; rather, I considered myself "stocky" because I had some muscle on my body. My legs were rather thick, but I thought they were still big from my days of playing soccer. My wife, Gail, now points out that, in fact, I was fat, and she loves to show my "fat pictures". Not only do I look fat in those pictures, but I also look unhealthy. At that point in my life, I thought I was eating fairly well. In hindsight, my diet was absolutely terrible, and completely different from the way I eat today.

The first step I took towards better health was in my early 40s, after I read a book about trans fats. At that time, I was a huge consumer of ice cream, thinking it wasn't a bad food because it contained natural ingredients, like cream and sugar. I remember a time when there was a huge sale on Edy's Ice Cream at a local grocery store – buy one, get two free. I was so excited, I managed to clean out the entire grocery store freezer and took home 27 half-gallon containers. Of course, I ate them all! Later, after reading the book about trans fats and learning how harmful they are, I wrote a letter to Edy's ice cream, expressing my dissatisfaction with the trans-fat content in their ice cream. How did they respond? Well, there was no letter thanking me for being a loyal customer, or for voicing my concerns. They just sent me coupons for free ice cream. So, what did I do? I went to the store and picked up more ice cream – it was free, what was I supposed to do? Another time, I asked the owner of a local Mexican restaurant to show me the oil he was using to fry his food. He brought out a large container labeled "partially hydrogenated vegetable oil". I proceeded to lecture him on how that oil is very harmful to his customers. The next time I saw him, he said that he tried to switch oils, but the other oils burned at high temperatures, so he went back to the old oil. Even though I enjoyed the food there, I stopped eating at that restaurant. I popped in a few months later to see how the owner was doing and found out that he was out of business. Hopefully, it wasn't because of me!

So, I started paying attention to food ingredients. But my big wakeup call came when my younger brother, Anthony, who was 41 at the time, was diagnosed with colorectal cancer. I still remember our phone call. I was shocked and terrified for him. Fortunately, after surgery, radiation, and chemotherapy, Anthony experienced a full recovery. But this just hit way too close to home for me. I was 44 at the time and believed that cancer was a random disease that anyone could get, and if there was a family history of cancer, you had a greater chance of getting it. I had no idea then that diet, accumulation of toxins in the body, living a sedentary lifestyle, constant stress, and lack of proper sleep can all contribute to getting cancer and other degenerative diseases. When my father was in his 60s, he suffered from angina, high blood pressure, and elevated cholesterol. At that time, I thought I was destined to follow in my father's footsteps with high blood pressure, elevated cholesterol, and blocked arteries, and that I would need to be on medications for the rest of my life. Again, I believed that, if there was a family history of disease, it was embedded in your DNA, and there was nothing you could do about it. I also believed that as you aged, it was natural for your body to break down.

So, in my younger years, these were my beliefs about health and aging:

- As you age, it is natural to put on weight.
- You could lose weight by simply exercising more.
- If your parents have heart disease, (or any other disease), you are bound to get it too.
- As you age, it is natural for your body to break down.
- All degenerative diseases, including cancer, are totally random (or hereditary) – you were lucky if it skipped over you, and unlucky if it didn't.

After educating myself extensively on health and wellness, I no longer maintain these erroneous beliefs.

As I mentioned, my wake-up call came in 2010, when I learned my brother was diagnosed with cancer, and I realized I was not invincible. I knew that if I didn't make changes to my diet, exercise, sleep, and stress levels, I could be heading down the same path. I had to take control of my health immediately. So, I started to educate myself by watching documentaries, reading books and newsletters, and immersing myself in anything I could get my hands on to learn about improving my health and avoiding disease. It became a passion and an obsession.

My first step to a healthier lifestyle started with Netflix. I watched the movie, "Fat, Sick, and Nearly Dead," a documentary by Joe Cross, who went through many changes of his own after his health was suffering. I followed the movie's advice and bought a juicer. My wife, Gail, and I "juiced" for several days, but had to stop because we both had constant diarrhea. We concluded that this type of dieting was too extreme for us, but when I look back now, I realize that we probably had diarrhea because we were juicing three meals a day! The good news is that the experience kick-started me towards eating a better diet. I also watched other documentaries on Netflix, such as "Forks over Knives," "Food Matters," and "Hungry for Change," each of which I highly recommend. I started to realize the strong impact that food has on one's overall health. Slowly, over time, I changed my diet, first eliminating all soda, then eventually eliminating ice cream, potato chips, and pretzels. As I eliminated foods, I added more fruits and vegetables. I continued to improve my diet and continued to work out. I replaced unhealthy, calorie-dense, and nutrient-deficient foods with healthier, nutrient-rich foods, and found that I did not miss the unhealthy foods. I switched over to non-GMO, organic foods. As my diet improved, I began to lose weight. While the weight loss was gradual, unlike what usually happens with most diets - which rarely work - I kept the weight off. I got down to around 168-170 pounds, and then plateaued. I was still happy with these results; this was my weight when I graduated college over 20 years earlier, a weight I thought I would never see again.

Because of the documentary movies I was watching, I started to adopt a partially vegan lifestyle. I removed all dairy and animal protein (except for wild-caught fish) from my diet. Later, I added back organic eggs and ghee (clarified butter). I continued to lose weight, and when I thought I couldn't lose any more weight, I made a few more changes to my diet and lost additional weight. This pattern continued about four or five times, until finally, I had lost 35 pounds. I now weigh 145 pounds, and this has become my ideal weight.

The more I learned, the more I was hooked on health and nutrition. I subscribed to Dr. Brownstein's "Natural Way to Health" newsletter. This newsletter contains extensive information on diet, nutrition, ways to improve your health and avoid disease, and the woes of the medical industry. I read every past and current newsletter in their entirety. Dr. Brownstein once believed what many physicians still believe today - that diet does not play a significant role in one's health. He explains that, while training to become a physician, he was taught very little about diet. Much of his training was spent learning to diagnose disease and treat it with drugs. He went through his own transformation from treating patients with drugs, to treating patients holistically with diet changes and supplements, and he experienced much better results. I have learned a tremendous amount from Dr. Brownstein's monthly newsletter, and I continue to learn and to tweak my diet and lifestyle in the process. For example, I have learned that many food products produced in the U.S., such as soy, are promoted as healthy choices, but are not truly healthy. For one thing, 90-95% of the soy produced in the U.S. is genetically modified. Apparently, the soy that we eat in this country is different from the healthier soy eaten in the East. The Asians eat Natto, Tempeh, and Miso from soy that is fermented, while the soy produced in the U.S. is not. Fermented soy is lower in anti-nutrient substances that can become toxic in the body and is easier to digest. It is also lower in phytates that prevent the absorption of minerals, such as magnesium, calcium, iron, and zinc. So, though soy is promoted as a healthy food, I would suggest avoiding it, unless it is organic and preferably fermented. Still, I would suggest eating it in limited quantities, as is done in Asia.

Food manufacturers, like pharmaceutical companies, are in business to be as profitable as possible for their shareholders. There is nothing wrong with making a profit, but when it comes at the expense of our nation's health, then something is seriously wrong, and needs to change. Food manufacturers produce "food" that can last on the store shelves for years. Many of these foods have little or no nutritional value and do more harm to the body than good. Many of these foods are also made from GMOs (genetically modified organisms), which Wikipedia defines as "any organism whose genetic material has been altered using genetic engineering techniques. The exact definition of a genetically modified organism and what constitutes genetic engineering varies, with the most common being an organism altered in a way that does not occur naturally by mating and/or natural recombination."[1] GMOs are also used to produce many medications, genetically modified foods, and other goods, and are widely used in scientific research. A wide variety of organisms have been genetically modified, from animals to plants and microorganisms. (GMOs will be discussed in detail in Chapter 12). I avoid eating all GMO foods, and recommend you do the same.

Similarly to my opinion of GMOs, I am not a fan of the diet industry. This massive, highly profitable industry peddles "diets" that simply do not work. Sure, you might lose weight if you cut portions and starve yourself, but eventually, you are likely going to revert to your old habits and gain back any weight you've lost, plus some. In addition, when the body is in starvation mode, it will access muscle for fuel even before it accesses fat, so starvation diets are not at all efficient in attacking fat stores. Furthermore, many diet companies sell very unhealthy food products, as is evident from their ingredients, which are typically loaded with added sugar and processed carbohydrates, fats, oils, and salt. Again, you might lose weight due to portion control, but the weight-loss normally doesn't last. In the long run, diets just don't work, and many are undeniably unhealthy. Over time, Gail and I started buying more and more organic foods, including fruits and vegetables, eggs, and meats. Interestingly, she was way ahead of me. When our children were infants, she bought them organic baby food and organic milk. Looking back, my kids were always smaller than most of the other kids in school, probably because the organic milk they drank did not contain hormones.

In addition to his newsletter, Dr. Brownstein has written several books, one of which is a good starting point for anyone looking to change their diet and improve their health: "The Guide to Healthy Eating," by Dr. David Brownstein and Sheryl Shenefelt. Dr. Brownstein has really opened my eyes to better eating and better health.

As I became more interested in health and nutrition, I expanded my knowledge about degenerative diseases, such as cancer, MS, diabetes, dementia, and Alzheimer's. Interestingly, although the books I read on these diseases were written by authors with different backgrounds, education, and training, all the authors have similar views and recommendations on living a healthy lifestyle. These recommendations include eating organic, non-processed whole foods, drinking adequate amounts of water, managing stress, getting enough rest and sleep, and reducing and eliminating toxins in the body. As I mentioned, there was a point in time when I did not believe that diet had any impact on one's health, and that developing a degenerative disease was purely random. But the reality is, unlike infectious diseases, which come into the body, degenerative diseases are created within the body. So, you don't "catch" cancer or diabetes, for example. These diseases occur because of a biological breakdown or an imbalance in the body and may take years or decades to develop.

So, what does "disease" mean? "Turning from health to disease, we know, of course, that conventional medicine deals with illness largely in terms of symptoms – tumor in the case of cancer, the aches and pains of arthritis, palpitations of high-blood pressure, gnawing pains of ulcers, etc. Rarely is much emphasis placed on causes, such as the individual's destructive life patterns, poor food, lack of sleep and exercise, constitutional weakness, or the damaging effects of the pollutants in our environment – all of which play a vital role in producing illness. For the most part 'curing disease' allopathically consists of attempting to alleviate symptoms, generally by means of a vast variety of drugs, or when deemed necessary, by surgical intervention or other biologically unsound means. Should any of these treatments result in the disappearance of symptoms even for the shortest period of time – the disease is deemed to have been 'cured,' even though the causative factors behind the symptoms have not been dealt with at all."[2] When it comes to degenerative diseases (often called "lifestyle diseases"), I truly believe there is a direct correlation to diet, exercise, stress, sleep, and the accumulation of toxins in the body.

The human body is a very complex and efficient organism that will do everything it can to function properly. But over time, if it is not properly taken care of, like a machine, the body will break down. Using a car as an analogy, if you never change the oil in your car, over time, that oil becomes gummy, and does not provide the adequate lubrication necessary for an engine to function properly. Eventually, the engine will break down. It's the same with the human body. If your diet consists of poor food choices, such as a diet high in carbohydrates, sugar, conventionally-raised animal protein and fat, and low in fruits and vegetables, healthy fats, and protein, then you are undoubtedly harming your body. First, your body needs nutrients, including vitamins and minerals, for proper functionality, and processed foods often contain little or no nutritional value. Instead, they contain processed carbohydrates, added sugars, highly processed oils, and processed (table) salt. Second, many of these processed foods also contain added chemicals that are foreign and toxic to your body. These toxins then need to be filtered out of your body, and if you overtax your body with these poisonous substances, you will overload your liver, whose job is to filter out contaminants from your body. If your body becomes overburdened with toxins, whatever cannot be filtered out through your liver, or other parts of your body, gets stored in your fat cells. In addition, whatever your body doesn't use for fuel gets stored as fat in the body.

Besides eating a poor diet, many people tend to lead a sedentary lifestyle. Just like a car that cannot sit for too long without being driven, the human body needs to move. Our ancestors spent much of their days moving, as hunter-gatherers or farmers. Over the past 100 years, things have changed a lot. There are less people doing physical work, like farming, and more people sitting at desk jobs. We also spend less time outdoors in natural sunlight, and more time indoors under artificial light. Consider my generation. As a child growing up in the 1970s and 1980s, I spent a lot of time outdoors (getting more sun in the process), playing unorganized games and sports. In the summer and on weekends, I would be outside the entire day, and wouldn't return home until dinnertime. So not only were we more active than today's younger generation, but we had less downtime for snacking. Now, consider my children's generation. They don't play as much outdoors, and often sit in front of a video game or on their electronic devices for hours at a time. Much of their socialization is through social media, not in person. Being indoors frequently makes snacking easier. Television has historically bombarded kids with ads for unhealthy cereals, snacks, and sodas and other sugary drinks. So, it's not surprising that, in this country, there is now an epidemic of childhood obesity and Type 2 diabetes (which used to be called adult onset diabetes). Given that sugar is highly addictive and very harmful to the human body, foods that are high in sugar, like cereals, cookies, snack bars, and sugary drinks, should all contain a warning label, just like cigarettes must contain warnings. Just how one cannot get lung cancer from smoking just one cigarette, nor will a person become obese or diabetic from eating one cookie. But over time, much like the results of regular smoking, carbohydrates, sugars, and other harmful food ingredients (like processed oils and fats, trans fats, artificial sweeteners and colors, and processed table salt) will cause harm to the body.

I am constantly learning and refining my diet and lifestyle, with the quest to have excellent lifelong health. Some would say that I am "obsessed," and while I don't totally disagree, I prefer to call it being "passionate." I try to share my knowledge with anyone who will listen to me, but, unfortunately, many people don't make their own health a high priority, or they just don't seem to care. Personally, I consider my health and the health of my family as the highest of priorities. As I said before, it takes a lot of effort to acquire and maintain good health, and it all starts with the food you eat. From the time spent on food shopping, to the preparation of foods in the kitchen, I admit, sometimes it can be a bit overwhelming. I know that many people may not have the time to prepare meals, so they end up picking up takeout or buying processed packaged foods. But even if it's labeled as "all natural" and organic, the reality is, if it comes in a box or a bag, that food is still processed. Moreover, at home these foods are often heated or re-heated using a microwave, and that can harm the nutrients contained in these foods. The bottom line is that eating well takes a lot of effort and dedication, but the payoff is your good health and well-being, so it is absolutely worth it.

Eating and Exercising While on Vacation

In 2015, my family and I went on vacation to Hawaii for 12 days. I was very much looking forward to a break from the routine and from work – I had been feeling burnt out at that time and needed the time off. I think it's important for your sanity to take a break from the stresses of life from time to time. Before we left for the vacation, we knew that the bills, work, headaches of life, etc., would be there waiting for us when we got back, but in the meantime, we were looking forward to getting away.

The first part of our trip was to Kauai, an absolutely beautiful island. While observing the local population, I noticed that many native Hawaiians were overweight. I was surprised and decided to go to a local breakfast hot spot to see what they were eating. The restaurant was packed with locals, most of whom were overweight. I was completely baffled by the menu. There were no healthy choices available. I ordered a sausage, tomato, and green onion omelet with hash browns. I was shocked when my plate was placed in front of me. To my disbelief, they served me sliced Vienna sausage out of a can, and a microwaved frozen hash brown patty. Without looking at the menu, Gail ordered the island's favorite breakfast special, the Loco Moco. To her dismay, it turned out to be a burger and rice smothered in gravy and topped with a fried egg, or in her words, "a heart attack on a plate." My son, Michael, ordered the fried steak, which looked inedible, and my daughter, Amanda, asked for fresh fruit, which they didn't have, so she decided not to order anything. In hindsight, we should have left after looking at the menu. The poor meal choices on the menu helped explain why so many native Hawaiians are overweight.

Next, we went to Maui, and though not as pretty as Kauai, the temperature was warmer, so we were able to do some sunbathing there. We ate some very good meals while in Maui, several times at the same restaurant for breakfast. This spot even offered the option of organic eggs at a slightly higher cost, which, of course, I opted for. I wish all restaurants offered this choice.

During this trip, though I strayed somewhat from my normal diet, I still managed to eat a good amount of whole foods, including fresh fruits and vegetables (we bought some fresh fruits and vegetables from several stands on the side of the road), and I ate a limited amount of refined foods. Amanda inspired me and pushed me to work out, so I worked out almost every day, in addition to the exercise from all the activities we engaged in. When I weighed myself upon our return home, I was happy to see I did not gain any weight while on vacation.

The point is, even when I'm on vacation, I try not to deviate too much from my normal diet and exercise routine. After working so hard at maintaining good health in my everyday life, it just does not make sense to go on vacation and revert to old (bad) habits. For one thing, I would probably feel lousy if I ate the unhealthy foods that I have given up. In addition, the further that I deviate from my normal routine, the harder it is to get back to my routine.

I know many people think, "well, I'm on vacation", and then use that as an excuse to eat the wrong foods, drink too much alcohol, and skip exercise. But the way I look at it is that, since I have made a commitment to myself to eat well and exercise, why wouldn't I continue to do that on vacation? If I've deviated a little from my normal routine while away, I go right back to my healthy routines as soon as I return home. I remain committed to eating well and exercising, even while away.

Eating and Exercising for Your Blood Type

I recently learned about a concept of eating right for your blood type. This concept is explained by Dr. Peter D'Adamo and Catherine Whitney in their book, "Eat Right 4 Your Type, The Individualized Blood Type Diet Solution". The book discusses how your blood type affects your dietary and lifestyle choices, and how to use that connection to help you achieve your very best health.

"The essence of the blood type connection rests in these facts:

- Your blood type – O, A, B, or AB – is a powerful genetic fingerprint in your DNA, especially when it comes to your diet.

- When you use the individualized characteristics of your blood type as a guidepost for eating and living, you will be healthier, you will naturally reach your ideal weight, and you will slow the process of aging.

- Your blood type is a more reliable measure of your identity than race, culture, or geography. It is a genetic blueprint for who you are, a guide to how you can live most healthfully.

- The key to the significance of blood type can be found in the story of human development and expansion: Type O appeared in our survivalist ancestors: hunter-gatherers; Type A evolved with agrarian society; Type B emerged as humans migrated north into colder, harsher territories; and Type AB was a thoroughly modern adaptation, a result of the intermingling of disparate groups. This evolutionary story relates directly to the dietary needs of each blood type today."[3]

Although high quality studies about this blood type concept have not been published, the absence of studies does not prove that it is ineffective. Furthermore, there may be some correlations between blood type and digestion, stress, and heart disease. For example:

- O blood types tend to have a higher level of stomach acid (hydrochloric acid) than other types, giving them the ability to break down animal protein better than other types, but subjecting them to higher risk for ulcers. Type As, on the other hand, tend to have the lowest stomach acid, making them more adaptable to vegetarian proteins. This lower stomach acid puts Type As at a higher risk for stomach cancer than other blood types.[4]
- Type As tend to have higher levels of cortisol, the stress hormone, in their bodies.[5]
- O blood types tend to have the lowest levels of heart disease, while types B and AB are at the greatest risk due to higher rates of inflammation.[6]

I have recently learned, through the help of a blood test kit that I ordered on Amazon, that my blood type is A positive. Interestingly, this may explain why eating dairy or meat causes me digestive issues, and why I fare better eating vegetarian proteins, including beans and grains. I've also learned that A blood types produce more cortisol, which may explain why I tend to suffer from anxiety and insomnia.

We've discussed how there are many diets to choose from, but most don't consider that different people have different nutritional needs and engage in different levels of physical activity. The "one size fits all" diet is simply ineffective. Contrarily, the blood-type diet separates diet and exercise into the four principal blood types, tailoring different regimens to specific body makeups. I will reference some of these concepts throughout this book, particularly in Chapter 8 (exercise) and Chapter 11 (diet). While I believe that no single diet or exercise program is right for everyone, I highly recommend their book.

Diet and exercise are only two of the ways that you can improve your health. In the following chapters, I discuss the things you can do today to improve your health tomorrow. I will start with some of the effortless ways to improve your health, leading up to the more impactful approaches that require more effort.

CHAPTER 3:
AIR OUT YOUR HOME AND YOUR OFFICE

According to the U.S. Environmental Protection Agency, (EPA), most of us spend about 90 percent of our time indoors.[1] The air in our homes and other indoor spaces is often more polluted than the outdoor air. Over time, the air in your home becomes stale and needs to be recirculated. The best way to clean the indoor air is to air out your home regularly, by opening your windows and doors. It is recommended that you do this every other day for 5-10 minutes.[2] If it is difficult to do this during the weekdays, make sure to do this every weekend for 30 minutes or longer, which is what I personally do. You might also consider getting an air purifier for your bedroom and other rooms. It not only cleans the air, but it also serves as a highly effective "white noise" maker. (I bought a GermGuardian Air Purifier on Amazon for under $100. Its triple filtration system claims to control and prevent the growth of bacteria, germs, and mold, and capture 99.99% of dust and allergens). It is also important to get an air purifier for your office if you can't open your windows. You may spend 8-10 hours a day at your office, and you should not have to constantly breath in stale, recycled air. If possible, whenever you are on a break, go outside to get some fresh air, especially on a nice day. You will also get the benefit of sunlight, as well. Speaking of sunlight, in addition to its other benefits, it also reduces harmful bacteria in your house. Sunlit rooms have about 50% of the bacteria of dark rooms.[3] So, open the shades and let the sunlight in!

Radon

While discussing indoor air, it is important to address radon. Radon is a colorless, odorless, and tasteless gas that occurs naturally from the breakdown of uranium in soil and rocks. Radon is found outdoors in harmless amounts. The problem is when this gas enters buildings and homes through cracks in floors and walls, construction joints, and gaps in foundations, and gets trapped inside. The highest concentrations of radon in the home are normally found in the basement or crawl space. According to the EPA, there are about 21,000 deaths from radon-related lung cancer each year. While this figure is nowhere near the 480,000 deaths a year caused by smoking, it's still significant. Radon is the leading cause of lung cancer in non-smokers.[4] Radon test kits can be purchased at home-improvement stores like Lowe's, Home Depot, or Walmart, or online at Amazon.com. It's best to test your basement and the lowest level of the home where people spend most of their time. If your home tests high, you may need to install a radon reduction system. Opening windows improves air circulation and ventilation and can help to move radon out of the house.

CHAPTER 4:
REDUCE EXPOSURE TO TOXINS

Unfortunately, the world we live in is full of many toxins. This includes the food we eat, the water we drink and bathe in, the air we breathe, the prescription drugs we take, the personal care and cleaning products we use, and other everyday consumer products. According to the nonprofit organization, Environmental Working Group, more than 80,000 different toxic chemicals have been released into the environment since the beginning of the industrial age. And every year, 2.5 billion more tons of chemical pollutants are added to the environment.[1]

In the human body, the liver is the main organ involved in the detoxification process. One of the liver's jobs is to keep the blood free of toxic substances. When the liver is functioning properly, toxins are removed from the body. But if the body becomes overburdened with toxins, the liver can become clogged, and lose the ability to detoxify the blood, leaving poisons to accumulate in the body.

In separate chapters, I will discuss contaminants in food and water, but in this chapter, I will focus on the other ways that we are exposed to toxins.

Cleaning Products

Many cleaning products contain harmful chemicals that can affect your health. Just read the labels on these containers. Some of these chemicals are known carcinogens. I highly recommend that you rid your home of these harmful products and use natural cleaning products instead. You can even use white vinegar or lemon juice for cleaning; both are highly effective, and non-toxic. Try to refrain from using air fresheners and scented candles; they, too, contain harmful chemicals. Consider using essential oils as a substitute. Fill your home with plants, which can help pull toxins from the air.[2]

Insecticides

Insecticides and herbicides made from toxic chemicals should be avoided at all costs. This includes Roundup, the most commonly used herbicide in the U.S. Roundup's herbicide glyphosate is a very effective chemical compound and is widely used by the industrial agriculture industry in crops, such as soy, corn, and wheat. GMO corn and soy, in particular, are heavily saturated with Roundup. It is also widely used by schools and many homeowners to control weeds. While Roundup may be highly effective at killing weeds, it may also be killing us. While the pesticide industry maintains that glyphosate is minimally toxic to humans, new research published in the Journal Entropy, written by Anthony Samsel and Stephanie Seneff of MIT, strongly argues otherwise. Dr. Seneff's study of Roundup's glyphosate concludes that this harmful toxin gradually disrupts homeostasis in the human body, resulting in disease and suffering. The consequences of months and years of exposure to glyphosate include:[3]

- Gastrointestinal disorders (gut bacteria are negatively affected by glyphosate)
- Obesity
- Diabetes
- Heart disease
- Depression
- Autism
- Infertility
- Cancer
- Multiple sclerosis
- Alzheimer's disease

You can easily create a natural alternative to herbicides, by combining vinegar, salt, and liquid dish soap. The acid in the vinegar and the salt are very good at drawing moisture from weeds. There is a horticultural type of vinegar that contains 20% acetic acid, which is four times the acetic acid contained in household vinegar, making it good for killing weeds, but should be handled with care. Another simple, natural option for killing weeds that grow in walkways is to boil a salt and water mix and pour it directly on the weeds.

Personal Care Products

You might not be aware that everyday personal care products, such as toothpaste, soap, shampoo, deodorant, makeup, lotions, and others, bombard your body with toxins. Beauty products, too, contain toxic substances, including an ingredient called "fragrance" or "parfum". Though they might sound harmless, fragrance and parfum contain an undisclosed mixture of potentially toxic chemicals. By law, manufacturers of body care products must disclose a product's ingredients, using the International Nomenclature of Cosmetic Ingredients (INCI) guidelines. But fragrance and parfum get a free pass under the law – the actual chemicals that make up parfum and fragrance can hide under those generic words. The Food & Drug Administration (FDA) exempts companies from having to specify the chemicals contained in parfum and fragrance, even though a product may contain synthetic, preservative, or allergy-provoking substances that you should know about. This loophole was created because fragrance is considered a trade secret. But this loophole comes at the expense of consumers' knowledge, and possibly their health. Take fragrance for instance. Although fragrance is listed as a single ingredient, in reality, it's often a blend of many ingredients. There are about 5,000 fragrance molecules that can be used to create a fragrance.[4] The chemicals contained in fragrances are absorbed into the body through the skin, and then into the bloodstream. Products that contain fragrance include perfumes and colognes, baby lotions and wipes, hand creams, air fresheners, candles, detergents, and dryer sheets, just to name a few.

More than 95 percent of chemicals in synthetic fragrances are derived from petrochemicals. These chemicals include benzene derivatives, aldehydes, phthalates, and many other known toxins that may cause cancer, diabetes, obesity, birth defects, nervous-system disorders, and allergies. In addition, studies have linked fetal exposure to autism, ADHD, and neurological disorders.[5] How does "fragrance" sound now as an ingredient in the body lotion you use every day?

"The disparity in standards between the EU and US has grown to the extent it touches almost every element of most Americans' lives. In cosmetics alone, the EU has banned or restricted more than 1,300 chemicals while the US has outlawed or curbed just 11. It's possible to find formaldehyde, a known carcinogen banned in EU-sold cosmetics, in US hair-straightening treatments and nail polish. Parabens, linked to reproductive problems, are ruled out in the EU but not the US, where they lurk in skin and hair products. Coal tar dyes can be found in Americans' eyeshadow, years after they were banned in the EU and Canada."[6] Unfortunately, the FDA has not been nearly as diligent. Because the FDA does not protect us, it is up to us to protect ourselves! Choose natural products that don't contain synthetic fragrances, dyes, triclosan, and phthalates. You can easily avoid synthetic fragrances by looking for products that clearly state what gives them their scent, or by choosing products that use essential oils instead. You can also opt for fragrance-free products; just be aware that, though some products claim to be "fragrance free" because they don't have a scent, they may still contain harmful ingredients.

Other Toxic Substances Found in Consumer Products

- **Bisphenol A (BPA):** The chemical, Bisphenol A, is used to produce strong plastics that are light and clear in appearance, as well as epoxy resins, which are used as adhesives. BPA is found in some water bottles, food containers, dental sealants, baby bottles, compact discs, cash-register receipts (always wash your hands after handling), floorings, enamels, varnishes, artificial teeth, nail polish, and parts of automobiles. BPA decays over time, causing it to seep out of the plastic and into the contents, such as into the water inside of plastic water bottles and into the food inside a plastic container. Bisphenol A is associated with many endocrine-related health problems, including breast cancer, prostate cancer, insulin resistance, behavioral changes, DNA changes, and obesity.

- **Phthalates:** This industrial chemical is used to make plastics and vinyl softer and more flexible. It is found in many consumer products, including cosmetics, personal care products (such as perfumes, shampoos, hairsprays), detergents, shower curtains, vinyl flooring, raincoats, food packaging, automobiles (excess gas causes the "new car smell"), and other products. It is also an endocrine disruptor, can affect human reproduction and development, and can cause cancer.

- **Triclosan:** This antibacterial chemical is found in many household and personal care products, including liquid hand soaps, toothpaste, shaving cream, hair products, cleaning supplies, and trash bags, to name a few. Triclosan is a known endocrine disrupter. Continual usage of triclosan may result in triclosan-resistant bacteria. It is best to avoid products that contain triclosan, especially liquid hand soaps and hand sanitizer.

- **Methanol:** This toxic alcohol, also known as methyl alcohol, carbinol, or wood alcohol, is used in industrial products, and is also the active ingredient in some hand sanitizers. Hand sanitizers containing methanol should be avoided, because when absorbed through the skin, it can be toxic or life threatening. Instead, look for hand sanitizers containing ethyl alcohol and/or isopropyl alcohol (also known as 2-propanol), as the active ingredient.

- **Polybrominated Diphenyl Ethers (PBDEs):** This chemical is a flame retardant, and is used in many household items, including clothing, carpeting, drapes, mattresses, furniture, computers, TVs, cell phones, and other electronic equipment. Some studies have found that PBDEs can act as endocrine disruptors and may affect the thyroid and liver.

- **Fluoride:** Fluoride is a naturally occurring mineral, found in water, soil, plants, the air, and in some foods, but too much fluoride in our bodies may cause health risks. This includes dental fluorosis, skeletal fluorosis, thyroid problems, neurological problems, and other problems. In 1945, Grand Rapids, Michigan became the first city in the world to add fluoride to its drinking water. Now, most of the tap water in the U.S. contains fluoride. Though fluoride was added to drinking water as a means to prevent tooth decay, it is debatable whether it actually helps in this regard. "The trend of decreased decayed, missing, and filled teeth over the past several decades has occurred both in countries with and without the systematic application of fluoridated water. This suggests that increased access to preventative hygiene services and more awareness of the detrimental effects of sugar are responsible for these improvements in dental health."[7] Many countries have removed fluoride from their water supplies, including some countries in western Europe. In addition to drinking water, fluoride is added to many toothpastes. I make sure to buy brands of toothpaste that don't contain fluoride, sodium lauryl, sodium sulfates, preservatives, artificial colors, artificial sweeteners, saccharin, propylene glycol, or gluten.

- **Bromine:** This halogen is toxic to the body and competes with the iodine naturally stored in your body. Excess bromine has been shown to cause iodine elimination in the body, resulting in iodine deficiency, which can cause problems for glands, including the breast and the thyroid. Unfortunately, our bodies are often bombarded with bromine, which is used in pools and hot tubs as a disinfectant and is also contained in pesticides. In addition, it is commonly used as a fire retardant found in many common consumer products, including carpeting, furniture, drapes, mattresses, clothing, computers, and electronic gadgets.[8] Bromine is also contained in some of the foods and drinks that we consume, discussed in Chapter 11.

- **Aluminum:** Another common toxin we are often unknowingly exposed to is aluminum. Though aluminum is naturally contained in some foods, like spinach and potatoes, it is often added to processed foods. It is also found in water, pharmaceuticals, vaccines, and antiperspirants. Many researchers believe that the use of antiperspirants containing aluminum increases the risk of breast cancer.[9] Because aluminum can be easily absorbed through the skin, you might consider avoiding all antiperspirants that contain aluminum. I buy deodorants free of aluminum, parabens, phthalates, and propylene glycol, and I avoid using aluminum foil for cooking.

- **Mercury and Other Toxic Heavy Metals:** Other toxic metals include mercury, lead, cadmium, arsenic, and nickel. All these metals can cause neurological issues and brain toxicity, which can lead to diminished brain function. One common, highly toxic metal that is lurking in many people's bodies is mercury. The main source of mercury exposure is amalgam fillings, which contain 50% mercury by weight. Mercury exposure has been associated with the following diseases:

  - Alzheimer's disease
  - Amyotrophic lateral sclerosis (ALS or Lou Gehrig's disease)
  - Autoimmune disease
  - Cancer
  - Guillain-Barre related illnesses
  - Multiple sclerosis (MS)
  - Parkinson's disease

So, how toxic is mercury? By law, dentists cannot flush an amalgam filling down the drain for fear that it will pollute the environment. Yet, the American Dental Association (ADA) claims that it is safe to put this toxic substance in our mouths. Studies have shown that the mercury in amalgam fillings can seep out of a tooth and be absorbed into our body.[10] Because this highly-toxic metal has no business being in our bodies, I went to a holistic dentist and had all my amalgam fillings replaced with ceramic fillings. If you decide to have your amalgam fillings removed, I strongly suggest that you look for a dentist who has the experience and the equipment to safely remove your fillings, limiting your exposure to the noxious substance. Mercury is also found in fish, discussed in Chapter 11. Mercury, when used as a preservative in the form of thimerosal, can also be found in multi-dose vials of flu vaccines.

Other Ways to Reduce Exposure to Toxins and Radiation

- Use stainless steel or iron pots and pans, instead of nonstick pots and pans.
- Limit your use of microwave ovens.
- Never microwave food in plastic, as it could seep into the food. The same caution applies to microwave popcorn and other packaged foods. Use a microwave-safe glass or porcelain container instead.
- Never boil food in a plastic bag.
- Don't keep water bottles in the car, since the plastic could heat up or freeze, and seep into the water.
- When speaking on a cordless phone or cell phone, use the speaker or a wired earpiece to reduce exposure to electromagnetic radiation. I know someone who had a cancerous brain tumor just above his ear. He spent countless hours on his cell phone for work, and he firmly believes his tumor was caused by cell phone exposure.
- Avoid keeping your cell phone in your pockets all day long. When not in use, keep it away from your body, including when sleeping, where it should be at least six feet away.
- Since you spend an average of 7-8 hours sleeping in bed, it pays to invest in a natural mattress and pillows, to avoid the toxins contained in most mattresses and pillows. These toxins include polyurethane

foam, formaldehyde, boric acid, benzene, and polybrominated diphenyl ethers, which are used as flame retardants. These chemicals are released as gases, which you subsequently breathe in every night.[11] I found a good, comfortable, affordable, and non-toxic mattress and pillows through Avocado Green Mattress, and I highly recommend them. The company is based in California, but they have a small showroom in Hoboken, NJ, where we tried out the mattresses and purchased one. The website is: https://www.avocadogreenmattress.com/.

Although it is impossible to eliminate exposure to all toxins, you can greatly reduce your exposure by eating an organic diet (Chapter 11), drinking clean filtered water (Chapter 9), using natural cleaning products, using natural personal care products, and investing in a non-toxic mattress and pillows. If you suspect that you have a toxin overload in your body, it is always best to work with a medical professional who is experienced in the detoxification and chelation process. This is not something that you should do yourself.

CHAPTER 5:
GET SOME SUNLIGHT

Just as plants need sunlight to grow, we need sunlight to thrive. Unfortunately, the media and the sunscreen industry portray sunlight as evil, insist that it causes cancer, and constantly warn us that if we go outside, we'd better cover up with sunscreen! Yes, of course, too much sun is unhealthy, a sunburn is harmful to your skin, and repeatedly getting sunburns can lead to skin cancer. But I have often wondered why people get skin cancer on parts of their body that never see the sun. While a lot of bad press links sun exposure to skin cancer, in fact there is plenty of evidence to the contrary. Believe it or not, melanoma is more common in areas of the body that are not exposed to the sun than in those areas that are. In 75 percent of cases, melanoma occurs on relatively unexposed sites.[1]

According to Dr. Joseph Mercola, a New York Times bestselling author, regular sunlight exposure lowers your risk of cancer and heart disease, and is the ideal way to get your vitamin D. All it takes to get a beneficial amount of vitamin D is 10-15 minutes in the sun at the peak of the day, and it is best to expose as much of the body as possible; of course, it is important not to burn. Vitamin D has many health benefits, but perhaps its biggest benefit is that it may lower your risk of dying from any cause. But what about skin cancer? "The bottom line: if you avoid the sun, your risk of vitamin D deficiency skyrockets. This will increase your odds of developing melanoma, as well as the two main causes of death, heart disease and cancer."[2] Because we are told to cover up every time we go outside, many people are deficient in vitamin D. In addition to exposing yourself to natural sunlight, it is still important to take vitamin D3 daily (D2 is synthetic and does not work as well), since most of us don't/can't get enough sun during the year. According to WebMD, "Low blood levels of [vitamin D] have been associated with the following: increased risk of death from cardiovascular disease, cognitive impairment in older adults, severe asthma in children, and cancer. Research suggests that vitamin D could play a role in the prevention and treatment of a number of different conditions, including Type 1 and Type 2 diabetes, hypertension, glucose intolerance, and multiple sclerosis."[3]

According to Dr. David Brownstein, vitamin D is a potent cancer preventer, it reduces cardiovascular disease, it reduces the risk of Type 2 diabetes, and it "has potent antimicrobial effects, which means that it kills microorganisms such as bacteria and viruses."[4] So, the sun is clearly one of those things that everyone should be exposed to in moderation.

Vitamin D is produced in the body when the ultraviolet rays from the sunshine contact the skin. The best time to be exposed to the sun is between 11 a.m. and 1 p.m., which is when the UVB rays are best for the skin to make vitamin D. UVA rays, on the other hand, penetrate the skin more deeply than UVB rays, and help us tan, but also cause our skin to age. Unfortunately, many people buy into the notion that all sun exposure is unhealthy, and that one needs sunscreen anytime you go outside. I strongly disagree. Again, just fifteen to twenty minutes of sun per day is a great way to get the vitamin D that our bodies need. Furthermore, many sunscreens contain harmful chemicals, some of which are considered carcinogens.

Given its vital role in your body's good health, it's important to test your vitamin D level from time to time to assure that it's not too low or too high. Determining your vitamin D levels is easy, and usually ascertained during an annual checkup. According to WebMD, the most accurate way to measure how much vitamin D is in your body is the 25-hydroxy vitamin D blood test.[5] If you test low, you should speak to your doctor about taking a vitamin D supplement (again, I strongly recommend the natural form, D3, and not the synthetic D2, but speak with your doctor about that as well).

In addition to lack of sun exposure, Vitamin D deficiency can also occur from a diet lacking in animal-based foods, such as fish and eggs (including the yolk). Obviously, animal-based foods are absent in a vegan diet, so if you are a vegan, it is especially important to take vitamin D3 supplements.

CHAPTER 6:
MANAGE STRESS AND ANXIETY

What is the difference between stress and anxiety? Stress is a response that occurs when we are overwhelmed by life's pressures, like a work-related issue, being pulled over by a cop, or a crisis at home. Stress causes a sudden release of adrenaline, which is a hormone that elevates our blood pressure and puts us in "fight or flight" mode. Anxiety is a reaction to stress, and causes our feelings of fear, worry, or uneasiness. Anxiety can continue even after the event that caused the stress is gone.

Constant stress can affect the whole body. "Chronic tension activates a stress mechanism which can overwork the endocrine glands and immune system, and lead to exhaustion and greater susceptibility to organ impairment and disease. One of the most serious consequences of this overactivated stress mechanism is that it cuts down on the efficiency of food metabolism and waste elimination. Even with a healthy diet, if the digestive juices are not secreted properly because stress has skewed the process, the body will have difficulty breaking down the nutrients into the microcomponents necessary for normal cell production."[1]

Stress is part of life; everyone experiences it. But negative thinking, outdated beliefs, and fear-based emotions all suppress one's immune system. Your thoughts affect every cell in your body. If unmanaged, stress can create imbalances in the body, and can often lead to disease. In fact, researchers have found that as much as 75% of our thoughts are negative, and that 75% of all illnesses are self-induced.[2] So, how can you manage stress? Physical exercise, deep breathing exercises, meditation, writing, reading, watching movies that make you laugh, getting sunlight, and being in nature are just a handful of easy ways to reduce stress.[3]

Physical Exercise

Regular exercise, including weight training, aerobic exercise, yoga, walking, swimming, and playing sports, can help manage stress. When you are focusing on your exercise or sport, it takes your mind off the stressors in life. We will discuss more about exercise in Chapter 8.

Hobbies

Hobbies, just like exercise and meditation, help get your mind off stressors, because you are focusing on something that you enjoy. It's never too late to start a new hobby or to learn something new.

Laughter

They say that laughter is the best medicine. In fact, studies have found that laughter raises levels of endorphins, the feel-good hormones that boost mood and reduce pain. Some benefits of laughter include:[4]

- Relaxation and decreased muscle tension
- Lowered stress hormone levels
- Reduced blood pressure
- Lessened perception of pain

Watching your favorite funny shows and movies can help you relax and put you in a positive mood, as can reading and listening to music.

Family and Friends

Connecting with family and friends can be a positive way to reduce stress and anxiety. We can gain love and support from our friends and family, and we can discuss the things that we are stressed about with them. If possible, hug someone (and your pet, if you have one) each day; this can make us and them feel good. In parts of the world where people live the longest, including Sardinia, Italy, Okinawa, Japan, Nicoya, Costa Rica, Ikaria, Greece, and Loma Linda, California, one of the common denominators - besides diet and exercise - is having familial closeness and a close social circle.

Deep Breathing

Deep breathing is vital for alleviating stress. "Focused, centered breathing calms down your mind, brings oxygen into your brain and cells, and releases poisons from the body. Many of us are constantly running around taking care of endless tasks, never stopping to quiet our minds. This tends to create shallow breathing, from the chest up, rather than abdominal breathing, which engages the diaphragm and allows you to take in oxygen more fully."[5]

Deep breathing is done by taking a deep breath through your nose and filling your belly with air (place your hand on your belly so that you can feel it rise). Breathe out through your nose (your belly should fall as you breathe out). Do this exercise for several minutes and you should start to feel more relaxed. I do deep breathing every night just before I go to sleep, and again in the middle of the night if I happen to wake up and can't fall back to sleep. I also do it during the day if I am feeling stressed or anxious.

Meditation

Meditation is a wonderful way to quiet the mind and reduce stress and anxiety. Most of us are rarely in silence, and meditation is a great way to find silence and peace in one's day. Studies have shown that meditation can create a state of relaxation that is the opposite of the fight or flight stress response. As it quiets the mind, meditation can help create health and balance in body, mind, and soul. There are many forms of meditation to choose from. You can find a professional for one-on-one instruction (which is what I did), you can join a group meditation class, you can find many guided meditations on YouTube, and you can read books and articles on the subject. I try to meditate when I can during the day, and again if I wake up in the middle of the night and can't go back to sleep right away. It helps to "quiet" the mind.

Tapping

According to traditional Chinese medicine, the body is composed of energy, and that energy can be disrupted by negative emotions and physical afflictions. Born from the principles of traditional Chinese medicine, tapping is an exercise that utilizes the body's energy meridian points to restore balance to the body's energy. While focusing on a simple mantra or positive statement about what is bothering you, you stimulate the body's meridian points by tapping on them repeatedly with your fingertips. Stimulating the meridians helps return positive energy to the body. I engage in tapping, along with meditation, to reduce stress and anxiety, and to help me relax, especially if I wake in the middle of the night and can't fall back to sleep. For more information on tapping, please visit https://www.thetappingsolution.com/.

Practice Daily Gratitude

Be thankful for the good things in your life. Practice gratitude daily to change a negative perspective. Write a list and place it where you can see it daily.

Sunlight

In Chapter 5, we spoke about the many benefits of sunlight. We can add reducing stress and anxiety to the list. The warmth and brightness of the sun help us relax. I usually feel the most relaxed when I am at the beach, or on my deck, on a warm, sunny day. In the winter, when the days are short and it is cold outside, many people, including myself, stay indoors and hibernate. About twenty percent of the population suffers from seasonal affective disorder (SAD), which is caused by lack of natural sunlight. Symptoms of SAD include depression, fatigue, carbohydrate craving, weight gain, and oversleeping. Exposure to bright light can help by resetting the body's biological clock, which can get out of phase with natural cycles of day and night.[6] To help me, I bought a Verilux HappyLight VT31 Lumi 10,000 Lux LED Bright White Therapy Lamp with Adjustable Brightness from Amazon for $39.95, and I highly recommend it.

A Word About Electronic Devices

Although electronic devices, such as smartphones, tablets, and laptops, have made life more convenient, they can also be major distractions to our everyday lives, since constantly looking at screens can add to our stress. "The combination of heavy smartphone and computer use further increases the risk of depressive symptoms, sleeping disorders, and stress."[7] For one thing, the blue light from handheld devices (and televisions) throws off the body's internal clock, or circadian rhythm, making it hard to fall asleep right after using these devices. Many people stay on their devices until late hours of the night, sacrificing adequate sleep. Furthermore, communicating with people on social media is not the same connection you get when you speak to people directly on the phone or in person. I used to let my smart phone control me. I had alerts on for all texts and emails and would regularly open Facebook so that I could view and "like" other people's posts. Doing this became a daily chore, and was creating more stress in my life, until I made the decision to mute my alerts, and limit my use of social media. I also now use the "Do Not Disturb" feature on my phone from 9 p.m. to 9 a.m., so that I won't be disturbed by any calls during those hours – other than those from family.

CHAPTER 7:
GET SUFFICIENT SLEEP AND REST

Sleep plays an important role in the body's health, particularly for the nervous system and the brain. Sleep gives the neurons we use in our waking hours a break and time to recharge, it improves our memory function, it helps us to regulate emotions and our immune system, and plays a role in growth and development.[1] But most of us don't get the recommended 7-8 hours of sleep per night. We avoid or postpone sleep to watch TV, read, play video games, work, surf the internet, and go on social media. It is very important to make sleep a priority and to have a sleep schedule. Stress and anxiety can also influence how much, and how well, we sleep.

As mentioned earlier, we know that watching TV and spending time on our computers or mobile phones before going to bed interferes with the body's circadian rhythm. "Your body evolved over time to sync to natural day and night cycles. Our ancient ancestors slept at night in darkness and stayed awake in the exposure of bright daylight. But today, many of us stay up late at night and use artificial light sources. That fools our master clocks into thinking it's day when it's actually night, and therefore it doesn't cue the sleepiness that guides you to get in bed."[2] So, exposure to artificial light in the evening can trick the brain to think it's daytime. Not getting enough sleep interferes with the healing process that takes place during sleep. It can also impair your memory, impair the ability to think clearly and solve problems, increase stress, and can lead to weight gain, a weakened immune system, accelerated aging, and many other health issues.

Many people suffer from sleep disorders. "According to the American Sleep Association, 50 to 70 million adults in the United States have some form of sleep disorder."[3] The most common disorders include:

- **Insomnia:** This is the most common form of sleep disorder. Some people have difficulty falling asleep, others wake in the middle of the night, unable to fall back to sleep, while others consistently wake too early. Insomnia causes fatigue, excessive daytime sleepiness, mood imbalance, lack of concentration, clumsiness, and serious accidents. General anxiety is the main cause, though some medications can cause or worsen insomnia.

- **Sleep Apnea:** If you are gasping for air, choking, or you stop breathing at any point while you sleep, there is a good chance you have sleep apnea. One in fifteen Americans are affected by sleep apnea, but it is most prevalent in overweight, middle-aged men and African Americans. While this disorder shares many of the same symptoms of insomnia, it can cause serious medical conditions. It is normally diagnosed through a sleep study and treated with a CPAP (continuous positive airway pressure) machine.[4]

Ideas That May Help for Trouble Falling or Staying Asleep[5,6]

- Have a routine to help you wind down before going to bed.
- Turn off all electronics an hour before bed.
- Wear amber glasses at night; they are orange-tinted and filter out blue light. There are also apps that filter the blue light from electronic devices.
- Remove computers and TVs from the bedroom.
- Keep cell phones at least 6 feet from your head when sleeping.
- Keep your bedroom dark and free of blue light. This includes digital clocks and night lights that emit blue light.
- Wear a sleep mask to further block out any light.
- Keep your room cool (60-68 degrees).
- Go to bed at the same time each night (preferably before 10 p.m., when you otherwise might get a "second wind").
- Avoid caffeine at night and, for those more sensitive to caffeine, stop consumption in the early afternoon.
- Drink caffeine-free tea before bed to help relieve stress and to promote a good night's sleep. Organic India Tulsi/Holy Basil Tea or organic chamomile tea are often helpful.
- Limit alcohol intake and quit smoking.
- Eat foods that promote sleep, such as leafy greens, avocados, walnuts, almonds, and cherries. Avoid foods that contain a lot of carbs or sugar.

- Don't eat within 2 hours of going to bed.
- Set the alarm for the actual time you want to wake up and skip the snooze button.
- Exercise often but do it earlier in the day – at least 4-6 hours before bedtime.
- If you take naps, limit them to 30 minutes, and take them earlier in the day.
- Use a white noise machine or use earplugs.
- Replace an old mattress.
- Meditate and do deep breathing exercises.

Sleep is something I struggle with frequently. I normally don't have trouble falling asleep, but I often have trouble staying asleep. I have a normal routine before I go to bed, which helps me fall asleep quickly. But in order to ensure that I get the 7-8 hours of sleep I need each night, I need to give myself a longer window of time in bed, so when I wake up in the middle of the night and have trouble falling back to sleep, I will still get enough sleep. If I don't get 7-8 hours of sleep, I am cranky the next day, and am not at my sharpest and best. I try to go to bed on weekdays around 10 p.m., so that I can be asleep by 10:30 p.m. at the latest. During the weekends, I normally stay up a little later. When I wake up in the middle of the night and cannot quickly go back to sleep, it is often due to anxiety. In order to reduce the anxiety, clear my mind, and get me back to the state of mind where I can go back to sleep, I go through a routine that includes tapping (described in Chapter 6), which lowers my anxiety level, and deep breathing and meditation, which help to clear my mind. I have also found that an air purifier makes a good white noise machine. I often take a melatonin supplement before going to bed. Always speak to your doctor before taking any medications or supplements.

In addition to getting enough sleep, it is important to rest. This is especially true if you are not feeling well or if you are feeling fatigued. On those occasions, your body is telling you to rest – listen to your body! There is nothing wrong with skipping a workout, or not participating in an athletic event if you are injured or not feeling well. This is the perfect excuse to watch TV, read, or just listen to music. In the summer, I often just sit on my deck or go to the beach to relax and soak up the sun. It is so important to balance activity and exercise with adequate sleep and rest.

CHAPTER 8:
GET UP AND EXERCISE

"That which is used – develops. That which is not used wastes away."

~ Hippocrates

"Walking is man's best medicine."

~ Hippocrates

In the previous chapter, I discussed the importance of sleep and rest. While they are crucial to good health, it is equally important not to rest too much – you need a good balance of rest and exercise.

Before we discuss the importance of exercise, let's first consider the results of sitting too long. A number of studies show that, even if you are very fit and work out frequently, sitting for much of the day puts you at a higher risk for dying prematurely.[1] Whether it's due to our jobs or leisure time, many of us sit for too long during the day. Our workdays consist of countless hours sitting behind a desk, as well as time sitting in our cars or in public transportation, followed by time sitting in front of our TVs before we go to bed. (The current 2020 pandemic, may be causing some of us to sit more than usual.) Our bodies were not meant to sit for this much time. We were meant to walk, squat, and kneel. Standing up every 15 minutes can offset the negative effects of sitting too long. This also helps your muscles stay strong and helps keep your circulation moving. There are plenty of available apps and fitness bands that can remind you to get up and move. If you drink enough water throughout the day as I do, you will make frequent trips to the bathroom, which also gets you off your chair.

Now, let's discuss the value of exercise and how it affects your muscles. Starting in your 30s, muscles begin shrinking, and they continue to weaken at a rate of .5% to 1% per year. "Study after study shows that people with less strength are more likely to be hospitalized or to die of any cause, including heart disease, stroke, cancer, and pneumonia, within a given period. Scientists haven't figured out all the reasons that strength predicts health and well-being, but it's not only because unhealthy people get weaker - in fact, a reduction in strength is a better predictor of dying from cardiovascular disease than is high blood pressure."[2] If you are told that becoming weaker is a normal part of aging, don't believe it. You can build and restore muscle mass and strength at any age, even at older ages.

Now that I hopefully have your attention, you should develop a formal exercise program with a routine you can stick to. Regular exercise can help your body function more efficiently. Your muscles, lungs, heart, brain, joints, and bones all benefit from regular exercise. For many people, finding the time to exercise is a big obstacle that holds them back. Yes, exercise takes time and effort - it is certainly easier to sit in front of your TV - but it does not have to take up a lot of your time. Even just 15 minutes of physical activity per day is beneficial to your health. Exercising regularly is very important and, like anything else, you may have to schedule the time for exercise to remain consistent. Once it becomes a regular habit, you will feel good and you won't want to skip it! Regular exercise can include:

Walking

This is a very basic, low impact, low effort form of exercise that most people should be able to do. It is suitable for any fitness level. This type of exercise can be done daily, as no recovery time is needed in between exercise. Some people prefer to walk alone, while others prefer to walk in pairs or in groups. Your daily walking can be done all at once or broken up into several shorter time frames. Walking can be done indoors or outdoors. The benefits of walking outdoors include breathing in fresh air and exposure to sunlight (as discussed in Chapter 5). Lastly, walking is free - all you need is a comfortable pair of walking shoes. So, if walking is a good way to get daily exercise, is jogging even better? Well, it depends. Jogging may burn more calories than walking, but it is also more taxing on your body. Brisk walking may actually have greater benefits than jogging. Because walking is a low-impact activity, you are less likely to experience pain or injury, as the load that you are putting on your body's joints is less than that of jogging. If you want to intensify your walking session, you can walk briskly and walk up hills. Walking is an easy exercise to stick to and do consistently.

High Intensity Interval Training (HIIT)

"All you need to do is look at nature for clues as to what an ideal type of exercise might be. Children and most animals in the wild do not run marathons or lift weights; they move at high speeds for very short periods of time and then rest."[3] I was always entertained watching my dog run as fast as he could for a brief period and then rest. This is the premise behind high intensity interval training, or what is referred to as HIIT. It is a cardio session of short, high-intensity bursts of exercise. In this form of workout, you push yourself for a short period of time, normally 30-60 seconds, then you rest or do a low impact exercise for 90 seconds and repeat. The entire exercise session may last only 20-30 minutes. It's the opposite of going for a long run, or riding a stationary bike, or jogging on a treadmill for 45-60 minutes. According to Dr. Mercola, "Traditional strength training and cardio exercises work only the aerobic process, but high-intensity exercises work both the aerobic and anaerobic processes, which is what you need for optimal cardiovascular benefit. With traditional cardio, you may not see the results you desire, even when you're spending an hour on the treadmill several times a week. While your heart is meant to work very hard and will be strengthened from doing so, it's designed to do so only intermittently and for short periods – not for an hour or more at a time."[4] This type of training can be done 2-3 times a week, but not on consecutive days, allowing your muscles time to recover. There are many sources of information about HIIT on the internet.

Strength Training

Gaining muscle through strength training (weightlifting or resistance training) will keep your muscles toned, help you lose excess fat, and help prevent age-related muscle loss. You should use enough weight to exhaust your muscles in fewer than twelve repetitions, but at least four repetitions; eight repetitions are ideal. You may want to do 2-3 sets of each exercise, but vary the exercises so that you work on the various muscle groups. This type of training should be done 2-3 times a week, but not on consecutive days, allowing the muscles time to recover.

Stretching

Many people live a sedentary lifestyle, leaving their bodies stiff, rigid, and pained. Regular stretching helps your muscles stay flexible and strong. Before exercising, it is a good idea to do some light warmup exercises and then stretch the muscles. After exercising, it is also a good idea to do some additional stretching. Yoga is a practice which incorporates stretching, as well as other physical movements, and provides great health benefits.

Exercising for Your Blood Type

What may be the right exercise program for one person, may not be the right exercise program for another person. According to Dr. Peter D'Adamo, each blood type has distinct exercise needs.

- **Type Os:** "If you are a Type O, you have the immediate and physical response to our hunter ancestors." Healthy Type Os need to release built up stress through vigorous and intense physical exercise. "Not only does a regular intense exercise program elevate your spirits, it enables Type O to maintain weight control, emotional balance, and a strong self-image." Recommended exercises for Type Os include aerobics, weight training, treadmill, stair climbing, martial arts, and competitive sports, to name a few.[5]

- **Type As:** "Type A often reacts to stress by mismanaging cortisol, which can cause weight gain, depress the immune system, and interfere with restorative sleep. Even at rest, Type A has higher levels of cortisol than the other blood types." Exercise should provide calming and centering experiences. For Type As, moderate isotonic exercises are recommended, such as hiking, biking, swimming, golf, tai chi, and yoga (for more calming exercises). This does not mean that you should not break a sweat. The important thing is that the exercise should be calming and not stressful. If you perform aerobic exercises, you should balance them out with relaxing, soothing exercises to best manage your Type A stress patterns.[6]

- **Type Bs:** "As a Type B, you confront stress very well for the most part because you blend more easily into unfamiliar situations. You're less anxious or aggressive than Type O and less physically impacted than Type A. Thus, Type B does well with exercises that are neither too aerobically intense nor completely aimed at mental relaxation." Recommended exercises for Type Bs include a combination of more intense physical activity, such as aerobics, tennis, martial arts, swimming, brisk walking, hiking, and weight training, and more relaxed exercises such as golf, biking, and tai chi, to name a few.[7]

- **Type ABs:** "Although we've seen again and again that Type AB acts as a marriage between Types A and B, in regard to stress, Type AB appears to share many of the same characteristics of Type O (fight or flight), along with a bit of overactive cortisol thrown in for good measure. Exercises that provide calm and focus are the remedy that pulls Type AB from the grip of stress." While calming exercises are recommended, it doesn't mean that you can't break a sweat. Recommended exercises for Type ABs include tai chi, yoga, golf, hiking, biking, brisk walking, swimming, and dance, to name a few.[8]

I have made exercise a priority in my life. Like most people, I lead a busy lifestyle, but I very rarely skip a workout. Because regular workouts are such a high priority to me, I don't schedule anything else during the time scheduled for my workouts. Of course, things unexpectedly come up, but when they do, I simply do my exercise session later in the day, or the following day. I work out on Sunday, Tuesday, and Thursday mornings, and each workout lasts about an hour, including time for stretching. So, my total workout time is only about 3 hours a week. Since I'm asleep for about 7-8 hours a night, I am awake roughly 110 hours a week. This means that my workouts take up only about 3% of my waking hours. When you break it down like that, the time I spend on these formal workouts seems insignificant. Do I enjoy working out? Not really, as the exercises aren't easy. But I feel good after each workout, and I look at each workout as an investment in my health, so I never want to miss it. About the only time I skip is when I am away (and don't have the opportunity to work out where I am), when I'm injured, or when I don't feel well enough to work out (but that rarely happens). In addition to my formal workouts, I also walk, and play tennis and pickleball (a cross between tennis and ping pong, and one of the fastest-growing sports). In the winter months, when it is too cold to walk, I jump on my mini trampoline.

I recently learned that I have type A blood. I continue to do weight training and aerobic exercise, but have cut down on the intensity of the HIIT exercises, which were causing me too much stress, so I have adopted a more moderate exercise program. I plan to add more calming exercises as well, and I plan to remain active and to exercise consistently for the remainder of my life.

Even if you have led a sedentary lifestyle and have not exercised regularly, it is not too late to get started. Begin slowly, by walking and stretching each day. When you are ready, start to incorporate more rigorous exercise and strength training (again, start off slowly and build it up). There are many apps that can track your exercise and movement. Each person's exercise needs will vary. It is important to check with your doctor before starting any exercise program.

Each decision that you make each day, whether to exercise or skip your workout, whether to take the stairs or the elevator, whether to take a walk or sit in front of the TV, will not only have an impact on your immediate health, it will also affect your future health. Join a gym (and actually go), take a yoga class, swim, take up ballroom dancing, or work out to an exercise video in your own home. Do it regularly and do it right away! Regular exercise is one of the best things that you can do for yourself. Exercise has been shown to improve many health conditions, and to be an effective treatment for depression. "It can tone the muscles and increase musculoskeletal strength; enhance stamina; improve oxygen intake; improve circulation, thereby bringing more nutrients to the cells and stimulating better waste removal; and decrease stress and its symptoms".[9]

CHAPTER 9:
DRINK PLENTY OF WATER

Water makes up 70% of the human body, and 80% of the brain. Water serves the dual function of delivering nutrients and oxygen to, as well as flushing toxins from, the body. So, it is essential to drink enough water to promote good health and optimal cell function. Good health simply cannot occur without adequate water intake. However, most people don't drink enough water each day, resulting in dehydration. Dehydration stresses the body and can lead to headaches and an acceleration of chronic diseases. According to Dr. David Brownstein, all chronic diseases exhibit some signs of dehydration, and all chronic diseases are accelerated by inadequate water intake. Many of the signs of aging, including the loss of elasticity of skin and muscles, are due primarily to the body's cells losing water.[1] It's also worth noting that, as we age, we have less water in our bodies, and we have a decreased thirst sensation, resulting in greater risk of dehydration among the elderly. The major symptoms of dehydration are thirst, dark-colored urine, dry and wrinkled skin, headaches, thinning nails, dry mouth, and fatigue. Because we all lead busy lives, and are distracted by work, electronic devices, and TV, we often don't drink enough water. Instead, we consume high amounts of soda, coffee, tea, and juice. These drinks contain substances, such as caffeine, sugar, and other items, that accelerate water loss in the body. Sports drinks are no better for you either. "Though by now most people are aware that sodas are laced with processed sugars like high-fructose corn syrup and artificial sweeteners, many don't know that their favorite sports drinks and vitamin drinks contain these sweeteners, plus a whole host of frightening extras: toxic chemicals like chlorine, fluoride, phthalates, BPA, and disinfection by-products (DPBs)."[2]

So, how much water should you drink? That depends on your weight and how active you are. A general rule of thumb is to take your body weight in pounds and divide by two. This number determines how many ounces of water you should drink daily. For example, if you weigh 180 pounds, you should drink 90 ounces of water a day, which is about six 16-ounce glasses of water. When you exercise, you may need more water, on other days, maybe less. It's important to listen to your body. When you are thirsty, drink water! If you haven't urinated for several hours, drink water! Sometimes, when you feel hungry between meals, you may actually be thirsty, so drink some water first. It's better to sip water throughout the day than to gulp it down when you are very thirsty. Start with a glass of water when you first wake up in the morning, and drink water throughout the day. The possible exception is just before, during, and right after mealtimes, because it's possible that water may dilute the acid in your stomach. Because there is conflicting information about whether you should drink water with your meals, I would suggest limiting the amount of water that you drink with your meal. In addition, you should avoid drinking large quantities of water before bedtime to avoid interruptions in sleep for numerous trips to the bathroom throughout the night.

As I previously mentioned, I used to drink a lot of soda. In fact, I believe I was addicted to it. But I was able to break this habit once I realized that, in order to lose weight and improve my health, I would have to stop drinking it altogether. Ending the consumption of soda is a great place to start for most people; cut out soda, sports drinks, and juices, and replace them with pure water. This one step will not only help you lose weight, it will start you on a path to better health. If it is difficult for you to transition from soda to water, you could start with natural carbonated water. If you find it difficult to quit cold turkey, then reduce your soda consumption over time, so that eventually, you will cut it out altogether.

What is the best water to drink? There are many sources of drinking water. You can drink tap water from your kitchen faucet, you can drink bottled water, or you can drink filtered water. Let's discuss all three.

Tap Water

Tap water in the U.S. is relatively safe to drink, but it contains trace amounts of many contaminants, including chlorine, fluoride, aluminum, arsenic, traces of prescription and over-the-counter drugs, and industrial waste products.

Bottled Water

Bottled water is marketed as superior to tap water. But most bottled water comes in a plastic bottle with a plastic cap, and that plastic can leach into the water you end up drinking. In fact, many bottled waters contain tiny pieces of plastic. In an analysis of popular brands of bottled water, the

World Health Organization (WHO) found that 90% contained tiny pieces of plastic.[3] In addition, many plastic water bottles contain bisphenol A and phthalates (toxic chemicals discussed in Chapter 4). A test conducted by the Environmental Working Group found 38 contaminants at levels similar to tap water.[4] "The bottled water industry really presents this image of purity, but our investigation demonstrated that it is really hit or miss, Environmental Working Group senior scientist Olga Naidenko, PhD, tells WebMD."[5] Though some bottled water comes from springs, much of it is no more than purified tap water.

Another major problem with bottled water is its negative impact on the environment. The U.S. is the largest consumer of bottled water in the world, consuming 1,500 plastic water bottles every second. These plastic water bottles end up in landfills, on sidewalks and streets, and in rivers and oceans. Approximately 46,000 pieces of plastic per square mile are floating in the ocean. This is killing wildlife and disrupting the environment.[6]

Filtered Water

There are many water filtration systems on the market, ranging from water pitchers to whole-house systems. There is also a big range in price for these systems. I have given a lot of thought to the different types of water filtration systems (water pitchers, countertop filters, and filtration systems that hook up to your kitchen sink), and I'm leaning towards a whole-house system, but they are expensive and have multiple filters that must be replaced regularly. For now, I have opted for an external refrigerator filter that connects to the water supply line. This filter gives my family access to pure drinking water and ice directly from our refrigerator. The filter is a Propur refrigerator water filter which, according to its website, removes over 200 contaminants, including chlorine, chloramines, lead, fluoride, PFOA and others. Unlike most refrigerator filters that remove taste only, this one removes contaminants. The filter is good for up to 9 months and costs $59.95. If you are handy, you may be able to install the filter yourself; otherwise, you may have to hire a plumber. If you buy this filter, ask the company to send you the metal fittings, which work much better than the plastic ones, or you can buy them at a home improvement store. To order this filter, go to: https://www.propurusa.com/Promax-Inline-Connect-Refrigerator-Filter.html. You might also consider getting a filter for your shower, to filter contaminants that would otherwise get into your body through your skin, or through your lungs, as you breathe in the steam.

Other Drinks to Consider

For some people, drinking enough water can be difficult, as they just don't enjoy it. Adding lemon, lime, or mint can certainly help, but you may still want more variety. You can drink vegetable juice (freshly made, not the pasteurized type), or drink a vegetable/fruit smoothie. Be sure to make your smoothies with lower sugar-concentrated fruits, like all types of berries, and not higher sugar-concentrated fruits, like mango and pineapple. Some flavored waters are OK to drink on occasion. I occasionally drink a flavored water made by "bai", which contains all-natural ingredients, but contains 55 mg of caffeine per an 18-fluid ounce bottle, about half the amount of caffeine in an 8-ounce cup of coffee. When I drink it, I normally mix it with water. Organic caffeine-free teas are another option. I enjoy "Dandy Blend", as well as some other organic teas. I don't drink coffee, but many people still need to have their 1-2 cups a day. If I drank coffee, I would drink organic, Swiss Water Processed, decaffeinated coffee. I also recommend using only natural sweeteners, such as stevia or xylitol. Alcohol should be kept to a minimum.

CHAPTER 10:
BALANCE YOUR GUT BACTERIA TO IMPROVE YOUR HEALTH AND IMMUNITY

"All disease begins in the gut."

~ Hippocrates

The digestive system is one of the most important systems in the body, yet it is often overlooked. The digestive system includes the mouth, salivary glands, stomach, pancreas, liver, gallbladder, and the small and large intestines. The gastrointestinal system contains more than 100 trillion microorganisms, some of which are healthy, and some of which are not. These microorganisms help us to digest carbohydrates, regulate metabolic functions, and produce multiple vitamins.[1] When the body's ecosystem is balanced, the ratio is about 85% healthy microorganisms and 15% unhealthy ones.[2] An imbalance in this ecosystem can result in constipation, diarrhea, gas, bloating, heartburn, poor digestion, and abdominal pain. Moreover, an intestinal tract that is imbalanced with unhealthy microorganisms will compromise your immune system and can lead to autoimmune and chronic diseases. Normal intestinal microbes regulate the immune system, since 80% of your entire immune system is in your digestive tract; the other 20% is made up of your skin and your lymph nodes. Your gut is also the second largest part of the neurological system, which is why it is referred to as the second brain. Your gut and your brain constantly send signals to each other.[3] This means that problems in the gastrointestinal system can cause issues in the brain and vice versa. So, what causes this ecosystem imbalance? It can be caused by poor diet (including a diet of refined sugars and carbohydrates, GMOs, gluten, dairy, alcohol, and caffeine), stress, chemicals, medications, and antibiotics. When you are anxious, you get "butterflies in your stomach," and it messes up your digestive system. Eating the wrong foods creates digestive issues, which make you feel anxious. For some people, this can be a vicious cycle.

The Benefits of Restoring Your Gut Flora Balance[4]

- **Obesity:** The makeup of gut bacteria tends to differ in lean and obese people. Studies show that gut flora is significantly less diverse in obese people than in people with normal weight. People are more likely to gain weight when their gut bacteria does not properly break down food, allowing their bodies to absorb more calories. If you are trying to lose weight, restoring balance to your gut bacteria is vital.

- **Depression and Anxiety:** As previously mentioned, the gut is considered to be your second brain. Serotonin, which is involved in mood control, depression, and aggression, is concentrated mostly in your intestines, not in your brain. Perhaps this explains why dietary changes are often more effective in treating depression than antidepressants.

- **Skin Issues:** Beneficial bacteria not only plays an important role in your gut health, it also plays an important role in your skin health. Eczema, which signals a problem in the immune system, can be improved by balancing the gut bacteria.

- **Cancer:** A 2013 study by researchers at New York University School of Medicine found that patients with colorectal cancer had a less diverse population of gut bacteria than healthy people. This may be because an imbalance of bad bacteria to good bacteria creates the conditions for disease to occur.

- **Colds and Flus:** May be reduced, or even eliminated, with a healthy and balanced gut.

Ways to Balance Your Gut Bacteria and Improve Your Immune System

- Eat a clean diet consisting of organic, non-GMO foods.
- Keep sugar to a minimum.
- Keep wheat to a minimum or, better yet, eat gluten-free.
- Keep dairy to a minimum or, better yet, eat dairy-free.
- Drink filtered water that does not contain fluoride or chlorine.

- Take antibiotics only when it is absolutely necessary.
- Don't use antibacterial soap or hand sanitizer containing triclosan.
- Eat foods that contain probiotics, which are an excellent source of beneficial bacteria. You should aim to eat fermented food every day, even if in small quantities. Not all probiotics are created equally. Yogurt, for example, is a great source of probiotics. But yogurt often contains added sugars, and is almost always pasteurized, which destroys the beneficial bacteria in the yogurt. If you eat yogurt, stick to the plain ones with no added sugar, and make sure it contains live cultures. You can always add fruit, nuts, granola, or honey to give it more flavor. There are also plant-based yogurt choices, such as almond, cashew, and coconut.

Foods That Contain Large Amounts of Probiotics

- Sauerkraut
- Kimchi
- Fermented vegetables, such as pickles, carrots, and beets
- Miso, tempeh, and natto, which are made with fermented soy
- Raw cheese
- Kefir
- Kombucha (make sure the sugar content is low)
- Apple cider vinegar

As always, it's important that fermented foods you choose are organic, raw, and do not contain any added sugars or vinegar (other than apple cider vinegar). If fermented foods don't appeal to you, then take a high-quality probiotic supplement containing multiple strains and billions of colony-forming units (CFUs) of bacteria. If you are taking antibiotics, it is especially important to take a probiotic pill, but it should be taken at a different time of the day than the antibiotic, as the probiotic bacteria could be destroyed by the antibiotic. Continue to take probiotics for a week or two after the course of antibiotics is completed. According to Dr. Joseph Mercola, choose a probiotic which has bacteria strains that can survive your stomach acid and bile, and make it to your intestines alive. "The probiotic activity must be guaranteed throughout the entire production process, storage period, and shelf life of the product."[5]

As I write this, the world is experiencing a global pandemic of the coronavirus COVID-19. This is a highly contagious virus strain, which poses an increased danger to the elderly and people with an already compromised immune system. According to Dr. David Brownstein, to reduce your risk of becoming sick with any viral illness, it is important to boost your immune system, which can be done by: eating a clean diet free of refined sugar, drinking enough water to maintain adequate hydration, exercising regularly, and taking vitamins A, C and D.[6] It also helps to get sufficient rest and sleep and to manage stress.

In order to maintain good physical and mental health, it is especially important to maintain a balanced digestive system.

CHAPTER 11: IMPROVE YOUR DIET

"Let food be thy medicine and medicine be thy food."

~ Hippocrates

Of everything discussed so far, I believe that diet plays the most important role in one's overall health and body weight. There have been numerous books written on the subject, with many opinions on what you should and should not eat. There are also many different diets, but no single diet is right for everyone. We are all different, and certain foods may be good for one person and not another; it all depends on your body's needs. Some people may choose a vegan or vegetarian diet, while others may choose to eat animal protein. In fact, some people might require animal protein in their diet, while others may not. According to Dr. Peter D'Adamo, and as touched upon earlier, this difference may have to do with a person's blood type. For example, people with Type A blood may thrive on vegetarian diets with plant-based protein, and not do so well with animal-based protein, while people with Type O blood, who have high levels of stomach acid needed to digest meat, may thrive on a diet high in animal-based protein.[1] So, each person's diet is unique to the individual. But I believe that everyone, regardless of their blood type, should eat a balanced diet with large portions of plant-based whole foods. I strongly believe that the food choices you make each day are some of the most important decisions that affect your present and future health. We all know that we should eat more fruits and vegetables and less processed foods, so common-sense rules. Food can either be your friend or your foe. Whole, unprocessed foods provide the body with the necessary vitamins and nutrients it needs to operate efficiently. Some of these vitamins and nutrients are used by the body right away, while others are stored away for future use. On the other hand, eating a poor diet consisting of processed foods can lead to many problems:

- Processed foods lack vitamins and nutrients, so if your diet consists primarily of processed foods, you are not replenishing the body's essential substances, and your body will use its own source of nutrients to maintain normal body function. Your body might even have to "borrow" from other parts of your body to get the vitamins and nutrients it needs, but it can do this for only so long. In the long run, eating a diet of processed foods lacking in vitamins and minerals will lead to poor health.

- Processed foods are loaded with chemicals that are foreign and toxic to your body. Your body must process these chemicals and eliminate them. This overloads your liver and other organs responsible for the elimination of toxins.

- If you eat a lot of high-calorie/low-nutrient processed foods, you will be constantly hungry, because your body is not getting necessary nutrients, so your stomach receptors are not signaling to your brain to stop eating. In contrast, when you eat high nutrient-dense foods, your body is getting the necessary nutrients it needs, and your stomach receptors are signaling to your brain that you have had enough. A good example of this is potato chips vs. almonds or other nuts. I used to be able to polish off a whole bag of potato chips in one sitting, but I can only eat so many almonds or cashews before I feel satisfied and don't want anymore.

Where to Start

Choosing the right foods can be a daunting task, especially if you are used to eating a diet consisting mainly of processed foods. When in doubt, think of our ancestors. They did not eat food out of a package – they ate whole foods that provided them fuel and energy. So, taking a cue from them, we should eat more plant-based whole foods and less foods made in a plant. Choose the highest-quality foods whenever possible.

Eating the Right Foods Means...

- Eating unprocessed whole foods, including fruits, vegetables, whole grains, healthy fats (such as avocados, olive oil, ghee, nuts and seeds), plant-based protein (such as legumes and beans), and some animal protein (such as organic grass-fed meat, organic poultry, organic free-range eggs, organic dairy, and wild-caught fish).

- Eating organic foods, although that's not always possible or affordable. At the very least, the food you eat should be non-GMO foods (discussed below).

- Eliminating processed "white foods" from your diet, including white sugar, white flour, and white (table) salt. This includes breads, pastas, cookies, cakes, pastries, etc. Highly processed vegetable oil should also be avoided.

- Eating most meals at home. Most of the food you eat should be prepared at home. This allows you to control exactly what goes into your meal and is less expensive than eating out. Typically, restaurant food is more processed and contains more sugar and salt.

Figure 12-1 below is an example of what a healthy plate looks like. In addition to the food categories listed inside the plate image, notice the non-foods that also nourish your body – such as relationships, physical activity, career, and spirituality, all of which play a vital role in your overall health and happiness.

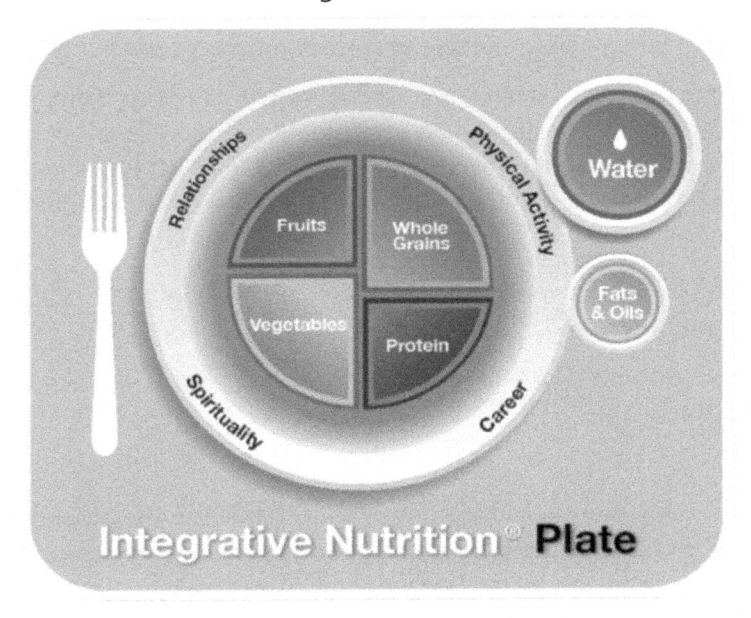

Figure 12-1

© 2013 Integrative Nutrition, Inc. | Reprinted with permission.
No further copying and/or republication is authorized.
Integrative Nutrition Inc. does not endorse the content contained in this book.

Eating Organic

There are many reasons for eating an organic diet.

- Organic farming precludes the use of synthetic pesticides, fungicides, and herbicides, all of which are used in conventionally grown food. Glyphosate, an herbicide, and known carcinogen contained in "Roundup", also destroys the beneficial gut bacteria.

- Organic food tastes better. I ate a non-organic watermelon and an organic watermelon in the same week and noticed a few things. In addition to size (the non-organic watermelon looked like it was on steroids), the flesh of the non-organic watermelon had a cracked appearance and a dull, lifeless color, while the flesh of the organic watermelon was solid, and had a more vibrant color. But the biggest difference was taste. Whereas the non-organic watermelon was very bland, the organic watermelon had a rich taste. So, not only is the organic watermelon better for you, it tastes much better too. There is a reason why the better-quality restaurants serve organic food – it tastes better!

- It's better for the environment. The chemical runoff of conventional farms negatively affects the surrounding ecosystem.

- It prevents soil erosion. Conventional farming damages soil at depths of 1-3 feet. "Even conservative estimates show that North American cropland is depleting soil at least 10 times faster than it can rebuild itself." It can take up to 100 years for one inch of topsoil to form.[2]

- It protects water quality. Conventional farming contaminates groundwater.

- It protects farmers and field workers from exposure to toxic chemicals.

Now, many people will maintain that organic food is expensive, which of course, it is. Indeed, my household food bill has skyrocketed over time. But, while I like to save money where I can, eating high quality foods is a top priority for me and my family. I would rather pay now for high quality food, than pay later, through health problems, co-pays, deductibles, prescription drugs, medical procedures, and time spent at doctors' offices and hospitals.

GMOs

According to NON-GMO Project, "A GMO or 'genetically modified organism', is a plant, animal, microorganism or other organism whose genetic makeup has been modified in a laboratory using genetic engineering or transgenic technology. This creates combinations of plant, animal, bacterial, and virus genes that do not occur in nature or through traditional crossbreeding methods."[3] GMO crops have been engineered to withstand the direct application of herbicides and pesticides. We've discussed glyphosate, the active ingredient in the common herbicide "Roundup", formerly produced by Monsanto, now by Bayer (which acquired Monsanto in 2018). With respect to glyphosate-tolerant crops (such as soy, corn, canola, sugar beets, alfalfa, and cotton), a farmer can spray these crops with glyphosate, which will kill the surrounding weeds without harming the crop. Consequently, GMO crops are responsible for the emergence of "superweeds" and "superbugs", which can only be killed with ever more toxic poisons, such as 2,4-D (a major ingredient in Agent Orange).

Some companies, like Bayer, and Monsanto before it, would like us to believe that GMOs are perfectly safe. But, despite biotech industry promises on this front, there is no evidence that any of the GMOs currently on the market offer increased yield, drought tolerance, enhanced nutrition, or any other consumer benefit. Furthermore, these companies continue to lobby against food labeling of GMOs. Just knowing this, how can anyone believe that GMOs are safe? If GMOs were safe, these companies would not have a problem labeling their foods as such. So, until it becomes mandatory for food labels to say that a food is genetically modified, if it doesn't say non-GMO, you should assume that it is probably genetically modified.

So, are GMOs safe to eat? It depends who you ask. According to Bayer's website: "[Genetically modified] seeds have been safety tested more than any other crop in the history of agriculture. Regulatory authorities around the world have concluded that GM crops are as safe for humans, animals, and the environment as non-GM crops."[4] On the other hand, according to the NON GMO Project's website: "There is no scientific consensus on the safety of GMOs. According to a 2015 statement signed by 300 scientists, physicians and scholars, the claim of scientific consensus on GMOs frequently repeated in the media is 'an artificial construct that has been falsely perpetuated'. To date, there have been no epidemiological studies investigating potential effects of GMO food on human health. Most of the research used to support the claim that GMOs are safe has been performed by biotechnology companies. A comprehensive review of peer-reviewed animal feeding studies of GMOs found roughly an equal number of research groups raising concerns about genetically engineered foods, and those suggesting GMOs were as safe and nutritious as conventional foods. The review also found that most studies finding GMO foods the same as conventional foods were performed by biotechnology companies or their associates. (Source: Center for Food Safety)"[5] So, you get an entirely different answer depending on whom you ask.

I try to avoid GMOs at all costs. First, GMO foods have been genetically modified, and we don't know the long-term effects of eating genetically modified foods. Second, these food crops are manufactured to be resistant to pesticides and herbicides, so farmers can spray these crops with chemicals (such as Roundup, which contains glyphosate, a known carcinogen), which kill the pests and weeds, but leave the crops intact. Though Bayer states that glyphosate is not carcinogenic, in 2019, a California jury found that Roundup weed killer was a substantial factor in causing a man's cancer and awarded him $80 million in damages. Apparently, there are thousands of similar lawsuits nationwide.[6]

Vegetables

Vegetables should make up the largest part of your diet and should be consumed daily. Sadly, for many Americans, this food group is usually an afterthought. Vegetables help move food along the digestive tract and clean your colon. Vegetables also have alkalizing properties, which reduce acidity in the body. Choose organic vegetables whenever possible. Organic vegetables are loaded with minerals, vitamins, and enzymes, which are necessary for the body to function properly. Most vegetables are best eaten raw, since cooking them can destroy their micronutrients and natural enzymes. Cooked vegetables do not nourish the cells as well as raw vegetables. If you do cook vegetables, use low heat and be careful not to burn them. Lightly steaming vegetables is a better option than boiling them.

Some of the most beneficial vegetables include:

- Green leafy vegetables, such as kale, spinach, and different types of lettuce (The dark ones are best; iceberg lettuce has minimal nutritional value.)
- Artichokes

- Asparagus
- Bok choy
- Broccoli
- Brussels sprouts
- Cabbage (green and red)
- Cauliflower
- Celery
- Chard
- Collard greens
- Cucumbers
- Dandelion and mustard greens
- Escarole
- Mushrooms
- Onions, including green onions or scallions
- Okra
- Parsley
- Peppers (green, red, yellow, orange, and hot)
- Radish
- Squash
- Watercress
- Zucchini

The great thing about these vegetables is that you can eat as much as you want. I know what you might be thinking; sounds boring. Yes, eating plain vegetables is not very exciting, but nobody said that they must be eaten plain. You can eat them with hummus, olive oil, lemon, or sea salt, just to name a few options. You can also blend them into a vegetable juice. Other common starchy vegetables, such as beets, carrots, eggplant, parsnips, potatoes, winter squashes, yams, and sweet potatoes, are also good choices, but should be eaten in moderation, since they have higher carbohydrate levels.

Fruit

Organic fruit provides many beneficial vitamins and minerals, but their intake should be limited, as all fruits contain sugar, some with a higher content than others. Fruits also serve the purpose of cleansing the body's digestive system. Some good fruits with lower sugar content include:

- Avocados (yes, technically a fruit)
- Berries (acai, blackberries, blueberries, cranberries, raspberries, strawberries)
- Cantaloupe
- Coconuts, including coconut flesh or unsweetened coconut milk (but not coconut juice or water, which has a higher sugar content)
- Guava
- Grapefruit
- Lemons and limes
- Nectarines
- Oranges
- Olives (also, technically a fruit)
- Peaches
- Tomatoes (also, technically a fruit)

Other good fruits to be eaten in moderation include: apples, apricots, bananas, cherries, grapes, honeydew, mango, melon, papaya, pears, pineapple, plums, pomegranate, tangerines, watermelon, etc., but keep these to a minimum, as they contain a higher amount of sugar. Dried fruit should be avoided or eaten in very low quantities, since they have a high sugar content. As nature intended, it is better to eat the whole fruit - such as an orange or apple, which contains fiber - than to drink its juice.

Grains/Carbohydrates

Carbohydrates are macronutrients that provide energy to your body in the form of calories. Your body turns sugar and starch into glucose, the body's preferred source of energy. Carbohydrates can be broken down into simple carbohydrates and complex carbohydrates.

- **Simple Carbohydrates:** These carbs have very little fiber and contain high amounts of sugar. This category of carbs includes processed white starches (like bread, pasta, cookies, crackers, cereal, bagels, white rice), white potatoes, fruit, and fruit juices. These foods provide a quick source of energy because your body can break them down quickly, but they are high on the glycemic index, and tend to spike your blood sugar level before it comes crashing down. When that happens, your pancreas needs to produce more insulin to regulate your blood sugar. A diet consisting of these types of carbs can lead to weight gain and increased risk of Type 2 diabetes. A diet high in simple carbohydrates will leave you hungry all the time.

- **Complex Carbohydrates:** These carbs contain plenty of fiber and lower amounts of sugar, and they take longer to digest and break down. This category of carbs includes whole foods, such as oatmeal, brown rice, sweet potatoes, yams, beans, whole-grain bread, and whole-grain pasta. Because it takes longer for the body to turn them into sugar, complex carbs supply a steadier source of energy. These foods are lower on the glycemic index, so they raise the blood sugar level slowly, and keep it stable for a longer period of time. Also, because these foods take longer to digest, you feel full for a longer period of time. These foods contain fiber, which mostly passes through the body undigested, and aids the body in the elimination process.

Grains are complex carbohydrates that contain a rich source of vital nutrients when eaten in their whole form, which includes the germ, the large endosperm, and the bran covering. Whole grains contain fiber, which helps with daily bowel elimination, and keeps the colon lining healthy.

For food manufacturers, processing extends shelf life, adding to their profits. But milling or processing grains, including the bleaching process, strips grains of their fiber and nutritional value. Unfortunately, many people's diets contain large amounts of processed grains, like bread, pasta, pizza, bagels, cookies, cake, pretzels, etc., that are made of processed "white" flour. There are several problems with this:

- Processed grains are devoid of any fiber or nutritional value.

- Many grains contain gluten, which is found in wheat, barley, kamut, oats (unless gluten-free), rye, spelt, triticale, and other grains. Gluten is what gives the elastic texture to dough. Unfortunately, gluten creates an inflammatory response in the body, especially in people who have autoimmune conditions, like celiac disease.
- Many grains, including wheat and oats, are often sprayed with glyphosate just before harvest. This process kills the crop one to two weeks before harvest to accelerate the grain drying process. (Organic grains are not sprayed with glyphosate.)
- Refined carbohydrates have a high glycemic index and, after ingestion, quickly turn to sugar, causing a spike in your blood sugar. Your body responds by releasing large amounts of insulin to regulate your glucose levels. This spike in glucose is stressful to the body and can lead to diabetes.
- According to Dr. Joseph Mercola, if your diet consists of a high amount of grains and sugar, you are conditioning your body to burn sugar as its primary fuel. "When you consume sugar or grains, your body stores the sugar in your liver and muscles. After the glycogen store is filled, any additional sugar that you eat is converted to fat for long-term energy usage. Foods high in sugar and grains will satiate your current hunger, but they will also set you up for metabolic disasters like obesity, fatigue, diabetes, and heart disease, and they fuel excess body fat and obesity-related diseases."[7]

Sugar

Who doesn't love sugar? Sugar makes just about any food taste better. It can also create a short-term "high," and be a quick source of energy for the body. Sugar itself, which is a carbohydrate, is not a bad thing. The problem is that many people consume large amounts of sugar, which can be highly addictive – studies have shown that sugar is as addictive or more addictive than cocaine.[8] Many foods naturally contain sugar, some more than others. With other foods, such as processed foods, refined sugars are added to them during processing. If a large portion of your calorie intake comes from sugar and grains, you are conditioning your body to burn sugar as its primary fuel. Sugar has a high glycemic index and is converted to glucose quickly after you ingest it. When you eat sugar, or other carbohydrates, your body releases insulin and leptin to remove excess sugar from the blood, allowing sugar to enter the cells so it can be burned as energy. If the glucose is not immediately needed for fuel, insulin will convert it to fat and store it in the body for long-term use. If you continue to eat a diet high in sugar and grains, eventually your body will develop a resistance to insulin and leptin, and you will require more and more of these hormones to do their job. Eventually, the body becomes "insulin resistant," causing constant hunger and cravings for sweets. Your body stops burning fat and, instead, stores more fat, especially around your belly. You gain weight, your blood pressure and cholesterol numbers climb, and you develop diabetes and other degenerative diseases.[9]

The Standard American Diet (SAD) consists of a large amount of refined grains and sugars, such as white table sugar, brown sugar, powdered sugar, turbinado sugar and high fructose corn syrup. Many of these sugars are hidden in processed foods under disguised names, such as:[10]

- Barbados sugar
- Barley malt
- Beet sugar
- Brown sugar
- Buttered syrup
- Cane juice
- Cane sugar
- Caramel
- Carob syrup
- Castor sugar
- Corn syrup
- Corn syrup solids
- Confectioner's sugar
- Date sugar
- Dehydrated cane juice
- Demerara sugar
- Dextran

- Dextrose
- Diastase
- Diastatic malt
- Ethyl maltol
- Free flowing brown sugars
- Fructose
- Fruit juice
- Fruit juice concentrate
- Galactose
- Glucose
- Glucose solids
- Golden sugar
- Golden syrup
- Granulated sugar
- Grape sugar
- High fructose corn syrup
- Honey
- Icing sugar
- Invert sugar
- Lactose
- Malt
- Maltodextrin
- Maltose
- Malt syrup
- Mannitol
- Maple syrup
- Molasses
- Muscovado

- Panocha
- Powdered sugar
- Raw sugar
- Refiner's syrup
- Rice syrup
- Sucrose
- Treacle
- Turbinado sugar
- Yellow sugar

It pays to be familiar with these names and to read the labels on all processed foods. If the food contains a high amount of carbohydrates and sugar, you are better off leaving it on the store shelf. As I said earlier, refined sugar has a very high glycemic index and is converted to glucose very quickly after consumption, which causes a surge in your insulin production. Another major problem with refined sugar is that it shuts down the body's immune system for up to five hours after ingestion, as it impairs our white blood cells, the first line of defense of our immune system.[11]

Like many processed foods, many drinks also contain high amounts of refined sugar, including high fructose corn syrup, which is two times sweeter than sugar. It is added to many processed foods and drinks because it is a sweeter and cheaper substitute for sugar. Unlike its response to sugar, the body has a difficult time using high fructose corn syrup as an energy source, resulting in excess fat storage. Again, excess fat storage leads to weight gain and other health problems.

Like many people, I used to eat a lot of processed carbohydrates and sugars. I regularly ate pasta, pizza, bread, bagels, pretzels, potato chips, sugary cereals, crackers, cookies, and other processed foods. That was also the period when I was overweight and had elevated cholesterol and triglyceride numbers. Looking back at my photos from that time, I appear bloated and unhealthy. Also, like many other people, I was under the impression that whole wheat breads and pastas were a much better choice than white breads and pastas, so I switched. However, I eventually learned that, while whole wheat flour contains some vitamins, minerals, and fiber, that does not mean whole wheat bread and pasta are healthier foods. That's because these food products are usually made with pulverized grains or flour, not whole grains. So, wheat bread, with a glycemic index value of 74, actually has about the same high glycemic index value as white bread (75).[12] The Glycemic Index ranks foods based on how quickly the body turns them into glucose, which creates the insulin response in the body. As stated earlier, higher glycemic foods get converted to sugar very rapidly, spiking blood sugar levels. Wheat also contains gluten, and while you may not have Celiac's Disease (which creates inflammation in the intestines), according to Dr. David Perlmutter, many people have sensitivities to gluten, which affects other parts of the body as well as the gut. Dr. Perlmutter believes that gluten and sugar can affect the brain and can even lead to Alzheimer's and dementia. Dr. Perlmutter points out that, even though our ancestors ate some wheat, it was not as large a part of their diet as it is today, where the average American consumes 133 pounds of wheat per year. In addition, the hybridized wheat that we consume today is quite different from the original, wild einkorn wheat consumed by our ancestors. For one thing, due to decades of agricultural changes, the wheat we consume today is higher in gluten than that in einkorn wheat, which has a much lower concentration of gluten, so it doesn't cause the digestive problems and inflammation of "modern" wheat.[13] On a side note, I recently had the chance to taste einkorn wheat bread, which is not easy to find, and found it to have a very rich taste.

After reading Dr. David Perlmutter's book, "Grain Brain" (which I highly recommend), I am now almost completely gluten-free. Although I do eat some gluten on occasion, such as pizza or bread, I keep it to a minimum. If you are going to eat wheat regularly, I would recommend eating Einkorn wheat (if you can find it), or sprouted wheat bread, which has some advantages over other whole-grain breads: it has a lower carbohydrate content, a lower glycemic index, higher nutrients, is easier to digest, and has a lower gluten level (Food for Life makes a 7-Sprouted Grain bread). If you are avoiding gluten altogether, some alternate grains to consider are:

- Brown rice
- Quinoa
- Buckwheat
- Amaranth
- Millet

It is important to note that, just because a food is labeled "gluten-free", that does not make it a healthy choice. In gluten-free foods, wheat is sometimes replaced with potato starch, rice starch, and tapioca starch, all of which also spike your blood sugar. So, even if gluten-free, it's very important to read the food label for its sugar and carbohydrate content. If you are going to eat pasta, there are several options made with brown rice, spinach and other vegetables, or beans, which are better choices than traditional white flour or whole wheat pasta. Pasta should still be eaten in moderation, especially if you are trying to lose weight or lower your blood sugar levels. Other substitutes for pasta include brown and wild rice, quinoa, and beans and legumes. I often make a vegetarian chili with beans and lentils, and eat it with brown rice, wild rice, or quinoa.

Before I improved my diet, I ate a lot of cereal, often for breakfast and after dinner, as a snack. Many of the cereals in the supermarket aisle are unhealthy, containing GMOs, processed wheat and other starches, high amounts of sugar and high-fructose corn syrup, and various artificial colors and flavors.[14] Again, eating these refined simple carbs can wreak stress on the body and lead to weight gain, insulin resistance, and diabetes. If you like cereal, try a low sugar granola instead. As a substitute for cereal, you can eat a bowl of berries (blackberries, strawberries, blueberries or raspberries), nuts and seeds (almonds, pecans, walnuts, pumpkin seeds, sunflower seeds, flax seeds), cacao nibs, and almond milk (all organic). I have found this combination of foods to be a much better choice than typical store-bought cereal, and this delicious meal contains protein, healthy fats, and little sugar, so it's an excellent way to start the day. Or I might have organic steel-cut oatmeal or non-dairy (almond milk) yogurt, to which I add almonds, pecans, walnuts, pumpkin seeds, sunflower seeds, or flax seeds. Though breakfast bars and protein bars are often marketed as nutritious food products, many include processed wheat, processed soy, dairy, processed oils, and high amounts of sugar. I am constantly looking for a tasty, healthy, and low-sugar bar; but so far, I have not found a good one that I can recommend.

As for other healthy snack options, I enjoy dark chocolate, and eat it almost every day. Chocolate is high in antioxidants and minerals. I typically eat dark chocolate consisting of 90% cocoa, which contains a low amount of sugar. Lindt makes a good bar. Although the Lindt packaging is not labeled "non-GMO," I contacted the company, and was told that they don't use GMO products in their chocolate. In addition, Lindt is a Swiss company, and GMOs are banned in Switzerland. Again, like other packaged products, it is very important to read the ingredients of chocolate bars since many chocolates often contain processed soy or a high amount of added sugar. Look for chocolate that has at least 70% cocoa or cacao, and does not contain processed ingredients, such as soy. Milk chocolate should be avoided, since it contains only 10% cacao, and high amounts of sugar. I also occasionally enjoy figs and dates, which are naturally sweet and contain no added sugar.

Artificial Sweeteners

In their efforts to lose weight, or to avoid gaining weight, many people choose low-calorie processed foods and diet sodas and other drinks. These foods and drinks are typically marketed as "sugar-free" and "fat-free"; but, they often contain artificial sweeteners, such as Aspartame (NutraSweet and Equal), Saccharin (Sweet 'N Low), and Sucralose (Splenda). According to Dr. David Brownstein: "Long-term use of artificial sweeteners can lead to a whole list of chronic illnesses, including obesity, diabetes, autoimmune disorders (including multiple sclerosis), thyroid problems, and cancer."[15] People are misled to believe that, if they eat sugar-free and fat-free food, they will lose weight. "The truth is that no artificial sweetener has ever been shown to reverse or prevent obesity. In fact, these substances trick the brain into thinking glucose is coming into the body. If glucose were ingested, it would result in leptin and other hormones being released to cause the brain to be satiated. When no glucose appears, a message is sent to eat more. Therefore, these artificial sweeteners actually make weight loss more difficult."[16] If you are looking for an alternative to sugar or artificial sweeteners, substitutes include raw honey, stevia, xylitol, and sucanat.

Fats and Oils

We are often told to avoid fat, particularly animal fat, to lower our risk for obesity, heart disease, and cancer. We have been led to believe that eating less fat and more grains and carbohydrates will make us healthier. But the reality is that, by following this misinformed advice, we have become the most obese people on the planet. As I mentioned earlier, two-thirds of Americans are overweight, and one-third are obese. This did not happen from eating fat. Eating fat does not make you fat; eating carbohydrates, particularly processed carbs and sugars, is to blame. Think about it - when farmers want to fatten up their animals quickly, they feed them grains, not fat. They know that eating grains will keep the animals constantly hungry and will fatten them up because these carbohydrates will be stored as fat.

Fat contains more energy than both protein and carbohydrates. It is essential for forming cell membranes and for hormone production, and it acts as a carrier for fat-soluble vitamins, such as vitamins A, D, E, and K. Fat tastes good and satisfies hunger.[17] "Fat is an important dietary component. In fact, every cell in the body requires fat for a variety of reasons, including helping maintain normal cell structure. Lack of fat will disrupt the functioning of the cell and weaken the cell wall. Fat and cholesterol are also necessary for hormone production. Lowering cholesterol will disrupt production of these hormones."[18]

Your body can burn either sugar or fat as its fuel. If you eat a diet high in carbs and sugar, your body will burn sugar first. When your body learns to rely on sugar as its primary fuel, you will likely feel a frequent hunger so that you can replace your sugar storage. With a constant intake of carbohydrates and sugar, your body has no reason to burn fat. One of the ways that you can teach your body to start burning fats is to eat more fats. But not all fats are created equally. There are good fats and bad fats. Good fats include omega 3s, omega 6s and omega 9s, and it is important to get the right balance of these omega fats in your diet. As humans, we evolved consuming a ratio of 1:1 omega 6s to omega 3s, but the average American consumes a diet with a ratio of 15:1 (or higher) omega 6s to omega 3s, leading to uncontrolled inflammatory responses.[19]

Good Sources of Fat

Good sources of fat include:

- Avocados
- Coconuts
- Olives
- Nuts and seeds
- Organic eggs
- Organic meat (poultry, beef, and pork)
- Wild-caught fish
- Organic butter and ghee (clarified butter)

I prefer ghee over butter, because the clarification process removes the milk solids, casein, and lactose, and I also prefer the taste over butter – it is a little sweeter.

Good Sources of Oil

Healthy oils include:

- Olive oil
- Coconut oil
- Palm oil
- Flaxseed oil
- Avocado oil
- Walnut oil
- Pecan oil

Because light exposure can degrade the quality of these oils, many of them are sold in dark bottles to keep out the light. If possible, choose organic, unrefined oils. When cooking with oil, use low temperatures, because high heat makes the beneficial compounds of oil start to degrade, and can make the oil harmful to consume. Some oils, such as flaxseed oil and extra-virgin olive oil, should be only used for low-heat cooking. Better choices for cooking include butter, ghee, coconut oil, and palm oil. I cook eggs in organic ghee or palm oil, and I use extra virgin olive oil in my salads and when roasting veggies. While these unrefined oils are better choices than processed ones, I would suggest consuming these oils in moderation. I also believe that it is better to eat the whole food than an extracted portion of it - such as eating the whole olive, instead of olive oil - as nature intended these foods to be eaten. I also eat plenty of avocados, which are wonderful in salads and as guacamole. For the most part, I have stopped eating tortilla chips and potato chips because they are fried in processed oils.

Bad Sources of Fat and Oil

Processed foods that contain fat typically contain unhealthy fats, such as trans fats or processed polyunsaturated fats, like processed vegetable oils (often sold in clear plastic bottles in the grocery store). These processed vegetable oils include soybean, canola, corn, peanut, cottonseed, safflower, and sunflower oil. These oils are highly processed with chemical solvents, steamers, neutralizers, de-waxers, bleach and deodorizers. They are high in omega-6 fatty acids, and a diet high in omega-6 fatty acids increases the risk of inflammation, cardiovascular disease, cancer, and autoimmune diseases.[20] These "dead" foods are typically made from GMO crops, are highly processed, devoid of any nutrients, and are very harmful to your body. These oils are often found in many processed foods, including cakes, cookies, crackers, salty snacks, and other packaged foods. In addition, you should avoid all margarines, and other so-called "healthy substitutes" for butter, including the numerous spreads sold today, because they contain processed oils and may contain trans-fats. All hydrogenated, partially hydrogenated, and trans-fats should always be avoided. Unfortunately, the FDA allows food manufacturers to label food "trans-fat free" if it contains less than .5 grams of trans-fats. Some foods and drinks contain brominated vegetable oil, made from bromine (a toxic halogen), discussed earlier in chapter 4. This vegetable oil should also be avoided. So, you know my mantra: always read the ingredients. If the food product contains any of these unhealthy oils, don't buy it!

Dairy, Why it is Best Avoided

Like gluten, dairy products often wreak havoc on the body, and are best avoided. First, milk, cheese, and other dairy contain casein, a protein that causes problems in people with leaky gut and gastrointestinal issues. Second, milk contains lactose, a form of sugar that many people are allergic to. "A milk allergy can manifest in many ways. The common symptoms are gastrointestinal problems, including diarrhea, bloating, gassiness, and constipation. However, there are many other symptoms related to dairy problems, including asthma, autism, behavioral issues, headaches, chest pains, dry skin, hives, rashes, stuffy nose, runny nose, and sneezing."[21] In addition, milk and most cheeses are normally pasteurized (heated to kill the bacteria), and this process destroys nutrients and enzymes, which aid in their digestion. Milk is often homogenized, the process of breaking up the fat globules in unaltered milk to extremely small particles to make the milk more uniform, which could alter how they act in the human body. In addition, much of the milk and cheese in the U.S. is produced by factory-farmed cows that live in crowded and dirty indoor conditions. These cows are typically fed GMO grains and soy (which affect their gut bacteria), are treated in an inhumane way, and are often given growth hormones and antibiotics. This is all ingested by the consumer.

Because of the allergies associated with milk, many people are switching to non-dairy alternatives, like almond milk or coconut milk, which my family has done for the most part. If you are going to drink milk, it is best to stick to organic, whole milk, since skim milk contains more casein.

Eggs

Because we've often been told that eating egg yolks raises our cholesterol levels, many people either avoid eggs altogether, or eat only egg whites. By doing so, they are missing out on one of the healthiest foods available - the entire egg. In fact, eggs are one of the most nutritious food sources, and they are one of the only foods that contains all the essential amino acids the body needs. But people avoid eggs because their doctors have instructed them to watch their cholesterol intake. According to Dr. David Brownstein, "The vast majority of cholesterol is produced in the liver. If you eat a lot of cholesterol in your diet, your liver will simply lower the production of cholesterol. Conversely, if you are eating a cholesterol deficient diet, your liver will pick up production of cholesterol."[22] Thus, your body requires cholesterol for different functions, and will produce as much as it needs. High blood cholesterol is an indicator of substandard health, and a sign that cholesterol is unable to enter the body's cells. Good health is the utilization of cholesterol, not its elimination. I eat 2-4 eggs a week, and always eat the entire egg. My cholesterol is perfectly normal.

At this point, you might be thinking, "but I thought animal fats are saturated fats that are bad for you and cause heart disease." According to Dr. David Brownstein: "Saturated fats have received a bad rap from physicians and dieticians as well as the media. In fact, we cannot live without saturated fats. My experience has shown that most people do not ingest adequate amounts of them. Optimal health is not possible without adequate amounts of saturated fats in our bodies. In order to digest and absorb protein in the diet, we need fat. Furthermore, mineral absorption is enhanced by fat in the diet."[23] In addition to animal fats, good saturated fats include coconut and palm oil.

Protein

Protein is the second most common substance in our bodies after water. Protein is essential to the body, necessary for building and repairing tissue, and is required for healthy muscles, skin, organs, the nervous system, and proper enzyme function. Adequate amounts of high-quality protein are necessary for good health, a good functioning immune system, and hormonal balance.

Animal Protein

Good sources of animal protein include:

- Fish: Fish is very high in protein and is a good source of many vitamins and minerals. Fish also contains omega-3 fatty acids, essential to the human body. Wild-caught fish is always preferable to farm-raised fish (discussed later). Smaller fish, like sardines and salmon, are better choices than larger fish, like tuna and swordfish, because they contain lower amounts of mercury.
- Eggs: Eggs contain essential amino acids and are an excellent balanced source of omega-3 and omega-6 fats. Eggs should be organic free-range, and the entire egg should be consumed.
- Poultry: Poultry contains amino acids and vitamins. It should be organic free-range.
- Red meat: Red meat contains the full complement of amino acids, saturated fats (essential to the human body), and minerals and vitamins, including B2, B6, and B12 (typically deficient in a vegan or vegetarian diet). It should be organic and grass-fed.
- Dairy products: If dairy is to be included in the diet, it should be organic from grass-fed cows.

Note: Animal protein tends to create an acid-like condition in the body. For this reason, animal protein should not be consumed in high quantities.

Plant Protein

Good sources of plant protein include:

- Beans, including black beans, pinto beans, navy beans, butter beans, cannellini beans, adzuki beans, black-eyed beans, chickpeas (garbanzo beans), kidney beans, red kidney beans, and soybeans (if organic and fermented)

- Legumes, including lentils, peas, peanuts, and alfalfa
- Grains, including oats, amaranth, quinoa, corn, spelt, teff, einkorn or sprouted wheat, barley, wild rice, sorghum, and farro
- Nuts and nut butters, including almonds, walnuts, cashews, pistachios, pecans, macadamia nuts and brazil nuts
- Seeds, including pumpkin, sunflower, sesame, flax, chia, and hemp
- Spirulina
- Nutritional yeast
- Vegetables, including broccoli, spinach, asparagus, artichokes, potatoes, sweet potatoes, and Brussels sprouts
- Fruits, including bananas, nectarines, blackberries, mulberries, guava, and cherimoyas

These sources of plant protein should be organic when possible, unprocessed, and never genetically modified.

Soy as a Source of Protein

Soy is marketed as a good, healthy source of protein, and is found in many processed foods, since it is one of the cheapest crops to grow and is widely available. But, the reality is that conventional soy is not a healthy food. There are several problems with soy:

- Currently, up to 94% of soybeans grown in the U.S. are GMOs.[24]
- Soy contains enzyme inhibitors that block the absorption of many minerals, including calcium, magnesium, zinc, molybdenum, manganese, and iron, which are essential to the human body. It can also cause deficiencies of vitamins B-12, D, E, and K.[25]
- Soy contains large amounts of phytic acid, which blocks the body's uptake of minerals in the intestinal tract.[26] Phytates are naturally occurring compounds found in plant-based foods, such as beans, grains, nuts, and seeds. Eating large quantities of soy and other legumes can result in low mineral levels.
- Soy adversely affects thyroid production, which can lead to hypothyroidism.[27]

- Soy is a goitrogen, which promotes the swelling of the thyroid gland (goiter). Graves' and Hashimoto's diseases, which are autoimmune thyroid disorders, have been associated with soy.[28]

Processed soy products include soymilk, soy cheese, meatless burgers, hotdogs, cold cuts, and tofu. Soy is often included in many processed foods including: bread and flour tortillas, cereals, cookies, crackers, cakes, chips, ice cream, protein bars and powders, instant formula, peanut butter, chocolate, margarine and spreads, dairy substitutes, vegetable oil, mayonnaise, salad dressing, and canned soups, to name a few. Because of soy's detrimental effect on the human body, even if organic, these processed products and foods should be avoided.

Soy can sometimes be hidden in foods under the following names:

- Glycine max
- Hydrolyzed vegetable protein
- Mono-diglyceride
- Monosodium glutamate (MSG)
- Tamari
- Textured vegetable protein (TVP)

I am not saying all soy should be avoided at all costs. There are healthy versions of soy, more common in eastern countries, that are a better choice, especially organic fermented forms of soy, such as miso, natto, and tempeh. The fermentation process helps to remove many of the naturally occurring toxins in soy. It also produces healthy probiotics in the soy. Still, it should be eaten in moderation. I eat organic tempeh or miso 1-2 times a week.

Food Allergies

While there are certain foods, such as processed foods, that should be avoided entirely, there are also foods that cause allergic reactions in some people. These foods trigger a response in a person's immune system, which recognizes some of the proteins in the food as harmful. In some cases, even exposure to a small amount of the food can trigger an allergic reaction and can be deadly. As they say, one person's food may be another person's poison. Allergy symptoms can include:

- Swelling of the tongue, mouth, or face
- Difficulty breathing
- Hives
- Rash
- Vomiting
- Diarrhea
- Anaphylaxis

While there are many foods that can cause an allergic reaction, the most common food allergies are:

- Wheat (gluten)
- Dairy (including milk, cream, ice cream, cheese, butter, and yogurt)
- Fish
- Shellfish
- Peanuts
- Tree nuts (e.g., walnuts, almonds, pine nuts, brazil nuts, and pecans)
- Eggs
- Sesame seeds
- Soy

Other common foods also cause allergic reactions in some people. For example, nightshade vegetables, which include tomatoes, potatoes, peppers, and eggplants, can cause an allergic reaction or intolerance. If you suspect a food allergy, it's important that you speak to your doctor. You can also try an elimination diet, in which you remove several suspected foods from your diet for a period of time, and then slowly reintroduce them, one by one, to determine the culprit.

Salt

Salt is an essential nutrient that is often vilified. Without salt, our bodies would not be able to undergo numerous and necessary chemical reactions, and we would not survive. But we are told that salt is bad for us because it causes hypertension. What many people, including some doctors, may not realize, is that not all salt is created equally. There is refined salt, which is not good for us, and unrefined salt, which is essential to the human body.

Refined Salt (Table Salt)

Your everyday table salt, found in many homes and in most restaurants, is put through a harsh refining process that removes minerals and leaves a final product with a bright white color. "Refined salt is a lifeless, devitalized product that has no minerals, leaving a product that is 99 percent sodium and chloride. The remaining 1 percent contains toxic additives such as ferrocyanide and aluminum."[29] The reason why this salt is refined is the same reason why foods are processed - for a longer shelf life, which, of course, increases profitability. "Refined salt is just such a devitalized product. Its use leads to a host of problems, including:

- Imbalanced pH (acidity)
- Mineral deficiencies
- Lipid abnormalities
- Cardiovascular disease
- Accumulation of toxic substances in the body"[30]

Unrefined Salt (Sea-Salt or Himalayan Salt)

Unrefined salt is salt in its natural state, containing over 80 minerals, which can differ among brands, depending on where the salt is harvested. These minerals are essential nutrients to the human body. Unrefined salt also helps balance the body's pH level, which is a measure of the acidity or alkalinity of bodily fluids. "The Benefits of Unrefined Salt include:

- Alkalizing agent (raises pH in the body)
- Balances blood sugar

- Helps relax the body for sleep
- Improves brain function
- Prevents muscle cramps
- Prevents varicose veins
- Prevents osteoporosis
- Regulates blood pressure (if adequately hydrated)
- Thins mucus"[31]

Unrefined salt is either pink or grayish in color, which comes from the minerals. Good sources of unrefined salt include:

- Alaea Red Hawaiian Sea Salt
- Bali Pyramid Sea Salt
- Celtic Sea Salt
- Eden Sea Salt
- Halen Mon Pure Sea Salt
- Himalayan Salt
- Krystal Salt
- Redmond Real Salt

If you have congestive heart failure or severe hypertension, it is imperative that you speak to your physician before adding any salt to your diet.

Processed foods, including packaged and canned foods, often contain high amounts of refined salt. Many restaurants, especially fast food and chain restaurants, also use high amounts of refined salt in their food, and often provide only refined salt on their tables. Knowing this, I often bring my own unrefined salt to restaurants. Although this may seem a bit unusual (as my brother jokes), it would be very unusual for me not to bring unrefined salt to restaurants.

Conventional Factory Farming

It's a shame that the government subsidizes big agricultural businesses, including large farms that use conventional methods of growing fruits, vegetables, and grains, and factory farms that produce beef, chicken, pork, and eggs. My feelings on this topic, and one of the reasons that I choose to eat little meat, stem from the horror I felt after watching a documentary depicting how the animals are treated in these factory farms. For those that can stomach it, the documentary is called "A River of Waste". It is appalling to see how these animals live in crowded, filthy indoor facilities, where they are literally on top of each other, stepping in their feces; many of these animals never see the light of day. In addition, they are fed grains and soybeans (which fatten them up), instead of their natural diet. The grains and soybeans fed to these animals are genetically modified, and totally alter the animals' gut bacteria, destroying their immune systems. Sometimes they are fed the ground-up meat of other animals. Because of their terrible diet and living conditions, these animals are often sick, so they are given antibiotics. In addition to the grains fed to these animals, to fatten them up as quickly as possible, they are often given growth hormones as well. So, when we consume conventional meat or other animal products, not only are we ingesting antibiotics and growth hormones, the composition contains a higher concentration of Omega 6 fats than Omega 3 fats. If you eat meat, it should always be organic, grass-fed, and pasture-raised whenever possible.

Fish, Farm-Raised or Wild-Caught?

I believe the term "farm-raised" was created to fool the public into believing it is a beneficial way to produce fish, but this could not be further from the truth. Farm-raised fish are raised in tanks, often under filthy conditions. These fish are fed grains and other foods that fish don't naturally eat, as well as antibiotics, and are often contaminated with PCBs (polychlorinated biphenyls). Farmed-raised fish have a higher omega-6 to omega-3 ratio than wild-caught fish. Farm-raised salmon are grayish in color and are dyed pink, so you won't notice the difference. In addition, a farm-raised fish tastes bland, so restaurants often coat it with some type of sauce to give it flavor. A wild-caught fish, on the other hand, tastes good all on its own. By the way, "Atlantic salmon", which sounds like it is harvested from the Atlantic Ocean, is actually farm-raised. Alaskan salmon, on the other hand, is wild-caught. When dining out, it pays to ask whether the fish is wild-caught or farm-raised before you order it. Though the waiter or waitress might not know the answer, the chef should know because they normally buy the fish. When I am dining out, I find out if the fish is wild-caught before I order. If it is wild-caught great, but if it's farm-raised, I won't order it. When in doubt, assume that it's farm-raised. Fast food restaurants and chains almost always serve farm-raised fish, whereas reputable local restaurants often serve wild-caught fish. Although wild-caught fish is more expensive, it is definitely worth it! Wild-caught canned salmon and sardines are a convenient and affordable option to eat at home. You can also find frozen wild-caught salmon in many grocery stores.

Dining Out

When you are watching what you eat, dining out can be a lot more challenging than eating at home. For one thing, you don't know what's in the food being served. In addition, many restaurants, particularly chain and fast food restaurants, add processed sugar and salt to the food they serve. Most fast foods contain refined carbohydrates, sugar, salt, and oil, and have little or no nutritional value. These foods overload your body with preservatives, dyes, synthetic hormones and antibiotics, and other toxins. Most fast food is also genetically modified. It's best to avoid fast food altogether. While I prefer to eat in non-chain restaurants, I occasionally dine at Chipotle, Panera Bread, and Cheesecake Factory, as they have decent food choices and better-quality ingredients.

Food Shopping

My main tip on food shopping is that it's best to buy most of your food from the perimeter of the store, because that's where you'll find the whole foods: produce, dairy products, eggs, meat, poultry and fish. It's the middle aisles that often contain the processed foods, such as cereals, cookies, crackers, chips, pasta, frozen foods, etc. My other suggestions on food shopping are:

- Choose one or two local food stores to do the bulk of your food shopping. These should be food stores that contain fresh, whole foods, preferably organic.

- Get to know these food stores well, and shop mainly from the perimeter aisles.

- Take the time to read the ingredients of all packaged foods. Don't just read the front of the packaging, which might say "all natural", "fat-free" or "gluten-free". Familiarize yourself with the ingredients by looking them up on the internet. Once you become familiar with the various ingredients, and you know what is safe and what is not, it becomes much easier to decide what to buy. By the way, the more ingredients the food contains, the more likely it contains harmful ingredients that you don't want in your body. Also, be aware of disguised ingredients. As mentioned earlier, there are 56 names for added sugars.

- A little-known fact is that the labels stamped on produce can tell you whether they are conventionally grown or organic. Foods containing 4 digits, beginning with the numbers 3 or 4, are conventionally grown. Foods with 5 digits, beginning with the number 9, are organic. Luckily, organic foods are labeled as such.

- Become familiar with the "Clean Fifteen Foods and Dirty Dozen" (see section later in this chapter).

- Do an inventory of food in your refrigerator and food pantry. Discard older foods or leftovers that have reached their shelf life to make room for new, fresh food.

- Make a list ahead of time of the foods you plan to buy. Better yet, create a list of foods that you buy often from each food store, and go through the list at home to see what you need. It helps to plan out the meals for the week. These meals don't need to be complicated.

My family does most of our food shopping at Whole Foods and Wegmans, but we also go to Costco and Walmart. When food shopping, be sure to stock up on the following:

- Lots of fresh vegetables, but don't overdo it, as fresh vegetables don't have a long shelf life. Once a food has ripened, such as when an avocado becomes soft, it should be refrigerated to last longer (see prior section on vegetables).

- A moderate amount of fruit, as fruit has a higher sugar content than vegetables. There is some higher sugar content fruit that you can eat occasionally, but mainly buy fruit with a lower sugar content (see prior section on fruit).

- Fermented foods (see Chapter 11)
- Complex carbohydrates (you may want to reduce or even eliminate wheat products; see section on grains, carbohydrates, and sugar)
- Healthy sources of fats and oils (see section on fats and oils)
- Animal protein (unless following a vegetarian or vegan diet; see section on protein)
- Plant protein (see section on protein)
- Unrefined salts and spices, which are wonderful to season and liven the tastes of foods (see section on salt)

Many of these foods are included on super foods lists. It's important to eat a variety of foods without overdoing it with any food. For example, if you eat a large amount of beans, nuts, and seeds, which contain phytic acid that binds certain essential minerals (calcium, iron, magnesium, and zinc) and reduces their absorption from food, you might become deficient in some of these minerals. One of my favorite foods is avocados. Avocados are one of the best sources of healthy fats available and are considered a superfood. Avocados can be eaten plain, with sea salt and pepper, sliced onto salads, chili, and countless other foods, or mashed for guacamole. If you only eat half of an avocado, refrigerate the half with the pit still inside (it will keep it from browning quickly).

It's best to eat mostly whole foods, but I do eat some processed foods on occasion, including foods packaged in cans (with BPA-free lining), bags, and boxes. Hummus, which is made from chickpeas or garbanzo beans, was once one of my favorite foods. I used to eat hummus almost daily, until I realized it was causing some gastrointestinal issues. Still, hummus is a great (processed) food choice for those who can eat it without issue. You can add it to salads, dip it with celery and carrots, eat it with crackers, rice, quinoa, broccoli, cauliflower, and even enjoy it on hamburgers.

Most people are on a limited budget and need to watch what they can spend on food. I, too, have limited funds, but I sometimes go overboard. For example, one time I went to Whole Foods and saw Steve Schirripa (who played Bobby Baccalieri on the Sopranos, and Detective Anthony Abetemarco on Blue Bloods); he was there to promote his pasta sauce, "Uncle Steve's". My daughter and I tasted the sample and thought it was fantastic, the best pasta sauce that we ever had. It contains all-natural organic ingredients, some of which are imported from Italy. It does not contain added sugars, as do many less expensive pasta sauces that load up on cheap ingredients, including processed sugars, oil, and salt. The sauce was on sale that day, so I bought 4 jars. Now, I only buy it occasionally or if it goes on sale, since it is regularly $9 a jar.

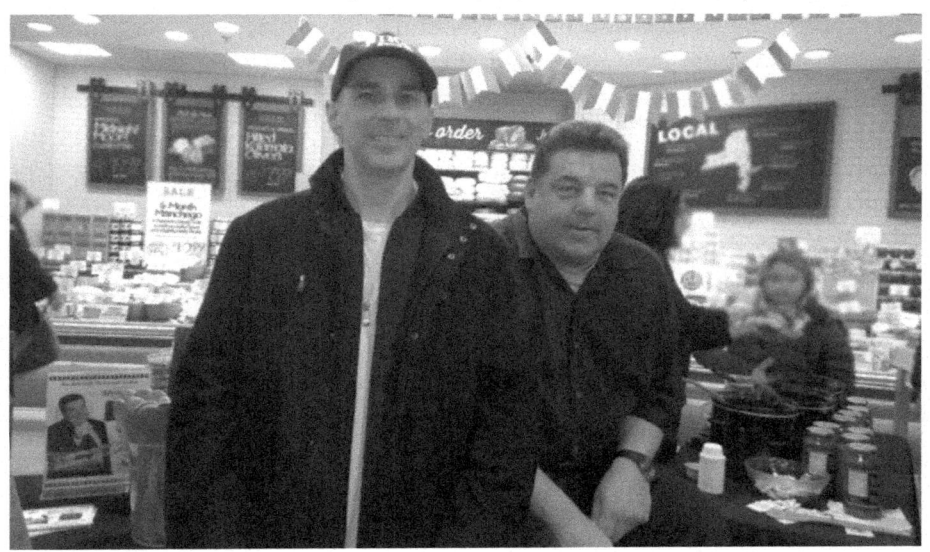

At Whole Foods, Marlboro, NJ, with Steve Schirripa

Both Wegman's and Whole Foods carry store-brand organic pasta sauces that are more reasonably priced than Uncle Steve's and are also very tasty. Now, you may be wondering, if I don't eat pasta, why am I buying pasta sauce? I occasionally eat pasta that does not contain any wheat or gluten. I buy pasta made with brown rice, beans, or peas, but again, only on occasion, as even these pastas contain a lot of carbohydrates at 46 grams per serving. One of my favorites is Wegman's Organic Green Pea Fusilli. But of course, you can put pasta sauce on other foods, such as steamed zucchini, squash, peppers, onions, chicken, hamburgers, ground beef, turkey, and of course, chili, which I make with lentils, several different types of beans, sautéed onions, and pasta sauce. Chili is an inexpensive meal, so I typically make a large pot and freeze half for another day. On occasion, especially when I dine out, I may eat pasta or bread, but at home, I avoid wheat as much as possible.

Back to food shopping. It does not have to be a chore. In fact, once you start reading the ingredients of foods, you will soon reach the point when you recognize which foods are safe to eat, and you will continue to buy those foods. Again, it bears repeating that the whole foods are normally found in the perimeter of the store, and the processed foods are in the middle aisles. Some food stores, like Wegmans and Shoprite, have organic sections, while other food stores have organic and non-organic foods mixed together. I find food shopping somewhat of an adventure. You never know what new foods you will discover. For example, when I realized that hummus was causing me gastrointestinal issues (and is not a good food for my blood type – discussed later), I looked for a replacement and found a very tasty almond-based dip called "Bitchin' Sauce". I started eating organic sauerkraut because the fermentation process of the cabbage preserves its nutrients and vitamins and creates beneficial enzymes and probiotics. But when I learned that cabbage is also not good for my blood type, I replaced it with fermented carrots and beets.

My family buys a good amount of organic vegetables, including lettuce, spinach, onions, carrots, celery, broccoli, Brussels sprouts, cauliflower, asparagus, and kale. For fruit, we buy blueberries, blackberries, raspberries, strawberries, grapefruits, apples, bananas, figs, and dates. Even though figs and dates contain more sugar than other fruits, they are still a better option than junk foods because they contain nutrients, vitamins, and fiber. Of course, the best fruit of them all is avocados; we normally buy 4-5 a week.

If you don't like cooking, there are companies that will ship prepared foods to your door. One that we like is Daily Harvest, which sells nutritious, delicious, clean, prepared meals that are delivered to you frozen. They offer smoothies, harvest bowls, soups, lattes, chia bowls, and oat bowls. Many of the ingredients are organic, and preparation is simple. To order, visit: https://www.daily-harvest.com/.

Clean Fifteen Foods and Dirty Dozen

Because it may not be possible or affordable to eat organic all the time, it is important to know which fruits and vegetables are the most and the least contaminated with pesticide residue. Here are the lists, according to the Environmental Working Group (EWG):

Dirty Dozen: These are the fruits and vegetable that are the most contaminated with pesticide residue, so it pays to buy organic:

- Strawberries
- Spinach
- Kale
- Nectarines
- Apples
- Grapes
- Peaches
- Cherries
- Pears
- Tomatoes
- Celery
- Potatoes

Clean Fifteen: These fruits are less contaminated with pesticide residue, so you don't always have to buy organic:

- Avocados
- Sweet corn
- Pineapples
- Sweet peas (frozen)
- Onions
- Papayas
- Eggplant
- Asparagus
- Kiwis
- Cabbage
- Cauliflower
- Cantaloupe
- Broccoli

- Mushrooms
- Honeydew melon

A small amount of sweet corn, papaya and summer squash sold in the United States is produced from genetically modified seeds. Buy organic varieties of these crops if you want to avoid genetically modified produce.[32]

I clean a lot of the produce that we buy with white vinegar, which kills germs. This includes fruits with skin that you don't eat (e.g., grapefruits and avocados), because, when you cut into these fruits, whatever is on the outer skin will get into the fruit.

High Sugar Impact Foods vs. Low Sugar Impact Foods

Many foods contain sugar and carbohydrates, and if you are looking to lose weight or to just improve your health, you will want to stick to low sugar impact foods for the bulk of your diet. However, there is often a lot of confusion about which foods have the highest sugar impact and which foods don't. A great resource on this topic is "The Sugar Impact Scales", which can be found at: http://jjvirgin.com/wp-content/uploads/2016/06/SUGAR-IMPACT-SCALES-JULY4TH.pdf.

Acidic vs. Alkaline Food

The human body attempts to maintain a healthy balance of acidity and alkalinity, which is measured as its pH balance. "pH" stands for "potential for Hydrogen," and is measured on a scale from 0 (the most acidic) to 14 (the most alkaline). Different parts of the body have different pH levels. For example, saliva has a pH level of 6.5-7.5, human blood is normally between 7.35-7.45, the upper stomach is between 4.0-6.5, and the lower stomach is between 1.5-3.5. Your lungs and your kidneys play a key role in maintaining a healthy balance of acidity and alkalinity. When your diet consists of many highly acidic foods, your body starts to become more acidic. Examples of higher acidic foods include processed foods (white rice, white flour), fried foods, sugary or alcoholic drinks, dairy and meat (particularly red meat). The most alkaline foods are most raw fruits and vegetables, raw nuts and seeds, and wild or brown rice. If you are eating the standard American diet of meat, sugar, and processed carbohydrates, your body will become more acidic. On the other hand, if you eat a balanced diet consisting of lots of fruits and vegetables, unprocessed grains, nuts, seeds, legumes, and less meat, you will have a more alkaline body. Why is this important? According to Dr. David Brownstein, most of his ill patients have an acidic pH level below 7. "Generally, the sicker the person, the lower (more acidic) their pH."[33] That's because it is believed that sickness and disease thrive in an acidic environment. According to Dr. Brownstein, unrefined salt, which is one of the most alkalizing substances, helps balance the body's pH level.[34]

Eating Right for Your Blood Type

As I mentioned in Chapter 2, according to "Eat Right 4 Your Type, The Individualized Blood Type Diet Solution", your blood type – O, A, B, or AB – is a powerful genetic fingerprint in your DNA, especially when it comes to your diet. Eating the right diet can help you naturally reach your ideal weight. The diet that our ancestors ate can be found in the story of human development and expansion:

- Type O appeared in our survivalist ancestors: hunter-gatherers
- Type A evolved with an agricultural, farming society
- Type B emerged as humans journeyed north into colder, harsher territories
- Type AB was a thoroughly modern adaptation, a result of the mixture of different groups.

This evolutionary story relates directly to the dietary needs of each blood type today. Because type Os tend to have higher stomach acid (hydrochloric acid) than other blood types, they can break down animal protein better than other types. Type As, on the other hand, tend to have the lowest stomach acid, making them better adapted to a more vegetarian diet.

People of different blood types have different gut bacteria. "This originated from our ancestors whose digestive tracts developed to accommodate one type of diet over another, and whose blood types controlled the ability to reject or co-exist with certain bacteria, but not others. Harmful lectins in foods can encourage the growth of problematic strains of bacteria, impairing absorption, damaging the intestinal lining, and causing 'leaky gut.' That is why the first line of support from healing your digestive tract and building a healthy microbiome is eating the right foods for your blood type."[35]

"Because the Blood Type Diet is tailored to the individual cellular composition of your body, specific foods will promote weight gain or weight loss for you, even though they may have a different effect on a person of another blood type. In that respect, there are no good or bad foods – just foods that are right or wrong for your blood type."[36] That said, as a person with blood type A, I find that I do better when I eat foods for my blood type, such as plant based foods. On the other hand, Gail, who is blood type O, has no trouble processing animal protein, but she tends to gain weight when she eats grains.

We know that eating the right or wrong foods has a direct impact on our health. But we are constantly bombarded with conflicting information. Much of our confusion is the result of taking the simplistic approach that one diet is right for everyone. So, what is the right diet? According to the book, "Eat Right 4 Your Type: The Original Individualized Blood Type Diet Solution", we cannot choose the right diet, it was already chosen for us many thousands of years ago.[37]

I highly recommend "Eat Right 4 Your Type, The Individualized Blood Type Diet Solution". This book makes it easy to understand which foods are best for each blood type, and which foods should be avoided. You might think that eliminating foods not right for your blood type would make your diet very restrictive, but that is not the case. As I have done, you can introduce new, ideal foods into your diet to replace the less-ideal foods. You might even discover that you like foods you never tried before. If you have gastrointestinal problems, like gas and bloating, a blood type diet may help you discover which foods are causing the problem. It may even help you lose weight, improve your elimination, and give you greater energy. But the book will not be beneficial unless you know your blood type. If you don't know your blood type, you can buy the Eldoncard Blood Type Test kit on Amazon and get instant results.

I believe that if you eat the right foods for you, you won't need to measure or count calories. I typically eat until I am satisfied, but not stuffed. After losing 35 pounds by changing the way I eat, I have maintained the same healthy weight for years.

Now that I understand the importance of a good diet, I eat a mostly clean diet. I used to try to be perfect, but now I strive to eat a clean diet 90-95% of the time (I occasionally veer off my diet, such as when I am on vacation or dining out). On occasion, I may indulge in a slice of pizza, a piece of bread, a beer, or ice cream. But I know that these foods are not good for me (and tend to cause digestive issues), so I return right back to my normal diet. If you are trying to lose weight, or if you have a health condition you are trying to improve through diet, maybe you cannot afford to "cheat" right away with foods that you should avoid. But the opportunity to indulge a little will come once you have reached your dietary or health goals.

A Sample of My Meals

I believe that eating well doesn't have to be complicated. I try to keep my meals simple, with little prep work. The last thing I want to do is spend countless hours preparing a meal, but that's me. Some of my meals can be prepared in 5-10 minutes or less, although there might be some initial prep work to prepare the food. With that said, here is my typical diet (most of the ingredients are organic and, if not organic, at the very least, non-GMO):

Breakfast

I usually start with some fruit, such as a grapefruit, or a handful of blackberries or other berries, with a few tablespoons of ground flaxseed. Or I might start with a smoothie made with spinach, berries or a half of an apple, and almond butter, plus one of the following:

- Steel-cut oatmeal (I will make 1 ½ cups on Sundays and refrigerate it for 3-4 breakfast meals.) To warm it up, I mix it in a saucepan with almond milk. I add unrefined salt, pecans, walnuts, almonds, pumpkin seeds, sunflower seeds, and cacao nibs (all organic). You can also add berries, or sweeten it with Stevia, Xylitol, honey, or a little maple syrup.
- Almond-milk yogurt with the above nuts and seeds, and berries
- "Cereal" made from a mixture of nuts, seeds, berries, cacao nibs, and almond milk
- Almond butter on an apple, on gluten-free Buckwheat Crispbread (made by Le Pain des fleurs), or on Sprouted Grain Bread (made by Food for Life).
- Two lightly fried eggs (cooked with ghee) on Thin Stackers rice cakes (made by Lundberg), with unrefined salt and organic, no

sugar added ketchup.
- Two lightly fried eggs, with lightly fried soy tempeh and unrefined salt.

These meals are low in sugar, high in protein and good fat, and loaded with vitamins and minerals. Notice I don't eat any of the standard American breakfast foods, such as processed cereal and milk, orange juice, waffles, pancakes, bagels, white toast, breakfast bars, breakfast sandwiches, muffins, doughnuts, etc., which contain large amounts of processed sugar and flour. I almost never eat breakfast out. I don't drink coffee, but may drink a cup of caffeine-free tea during the day or at night before bed. I normally don't drink much with my meals, except to take my daily supplements.

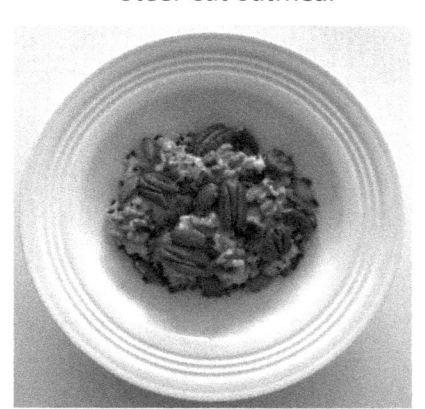

Steel-cut oatmeal

Lunch

I am truly fortunate to work a mile from my home, and to also work with Gail, so we often go home together for lunch. At lunch, I may heat up leftovers, or I will eat one of the following:

- A can of wild-caught salmon mashed with unrefined salt and avocado oil mayonnaise (made by Primal Kitchen). Sometimes I mix in fermented carrots or beets (made by Real Pickles), shredded broccoli slaw, or shredded carrots. I often eat this on "Jilz Crackerz", or on an almond flour wrap (made by Siete) or a brown rice tortilla (made by Food for Life), which are good alternatives to wheat wraps.
- Black bean dip (made by Better Bean), fermented vegetables, and Bitchin' Sauce (made by Bitchin' Inc.) in an almond flour or brown

rice wrap, with unrefined salt

- Mashed avocado with unrefined salt, on the crackers/wraps mentioned above
- Two eggs fried in ghee, with spinach, onions, or leftover broccoli/Brussels sprouts (see dinner section)
- Prepared Harvest Bowl meals (mentioned earlier)
- Dried seaweed from time to time, for the iodine

If I eat lunch out, I typically eat:

- A salad from Whole Foods – with olive oil and apple cider vinegar.
- A salad from Panera Bread – I add avocado and skip the chicken, cheese, and dressing and add olive oil.
- A salad bowl from Chipotle – I normally add brown rice, black beans, pinto beans, veggies, salsa, and guacamole. (Their guacamole is terrific!) On occasion, I order the chips with guacamole.

I used to eat a lot of subs, sandwiches, and pizza for lunch, as many people do today. These foods are not healthy and will surely make you gain weight. Speaking of pizza, I once thought it was a relatively healthy food choice. But the reality is, when you break it down, pizza is not a healthy food, and you will gain weight if you eat it often. Take a look at pizza by Papa John's, whose motto is "Better Ingredients, Better Pizza". Its website states that the Traditional Hand-Tossed Pizza is made from the following ingredients:[38]

- Fresh dough: Unbleached enriched wheat flour, water, sugar, soybean oil, salt, and yeast
- Cheese: Part skim mozzarella cheese, pasteurized milk, cultures, salt, enzymes, modified food starch, sugarcane fiber, whey protein concentrate, and sodium citrate
- Pizza sauce: Fresh vine-ripened tomatoes (our tomatoes are freshly packed from vine to can in the same day), sunflower oil, sugar, salt, garlic, spices, extra virgin olive oil, and citric acid (maintains freshness)

While the ingredients may seem OK to most people, both the dough and cheese are highly processed. And this list does not include any of the toppings, many, or all of which might also be processed. The point is that, while I applaud Papa John's for including their ingredients on their website, pizza, in general, is not a healthy food choice. In addition, if you are trying to lose weight, avoid pizza and other refined carbohydrates (discussed earlier) that are a large part of the standard American diet. If you like sandwiches, stick to whole grain bread, preferably sprouted, or wraps made from whole grains or almond flour. Deli meats should be organic with no added nitrates.

Dinner

At least 3-4 times a week, my entire dinner will consist of a huge salad. I typically open the refrigerator and pantry to see what we have available. This may include:

- Spring mix lettuce
- Romaine lettuce
- Spinach
- Kale
- Broccoli slaw
- Shredded carrots
- Celery
- Avocado
- Black beans
- Fermented vegetables (carrots or beets)
- Olives
- Hard-boiled eggs
- Sardines
- Artichokes
- Nuts or seeds

For dressing, I often mix some olive oil and Bitchin' Sauce, and then add unrefined salt. While I tend to eat a large salad, it is very nutrient-rich, and not a heavy meal.

We also prepare meals consisting of:

- Baked wild-caught salmon
- A vegetarian chili made with different types of lentils, black beans, pinto beans, onions, tomato sauce, and unrefined salt. I may also make brown rice, wild rice, or quinoa. I often eat ½ an avocado with the meal.
- Black beans with onions and spinach (sautéed in ghee), over quinoa
- Steamed broccoli and Brussels sprouts. Once steamed, I add olive oil and unrefined salt.
- Baked Brussels sprouts with olive oil and unrefined salt
- Steamed squash and zucchini with olive oil and unrefined salt
- Tempeh stir-fry with celery, broccoli, onions, and cashews
- Occasional gluten-free pizza or pasta

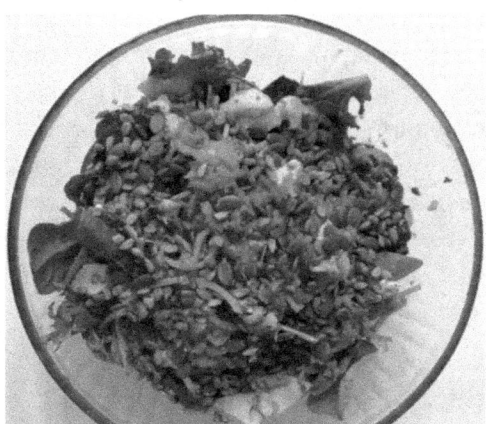

An example of a dinner salad

Stir fry

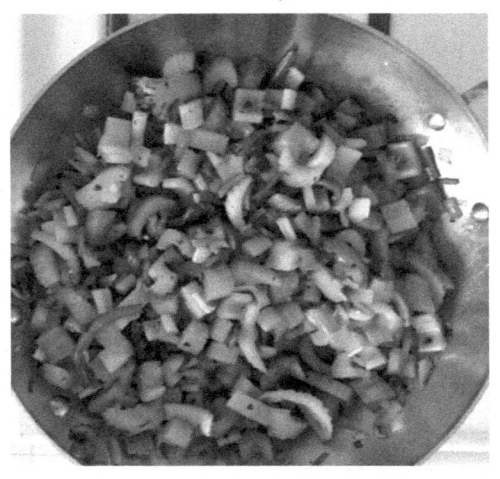

Snacks/Dessert

I like sugar as much as the next person, but I realize that, in order to maintain good health and not gain weight, I need to limit my intake. I normally eat the following as snacks or dessert:

- Dark chocolate: Dark chocolate contains antioxidants, flavonoids, and healthy fats, which have many health benefits. I eat two squares of Lindt 90% cacao dark chocolate almost daily (Lindt chocolate is widely available). I also eat Theo's Dark chocolate with sea salt and almonds. I normally eat chocolate in the early afternoon, as I am sensitive to the caffeine contained in chocolate. I avoid all milk chocolate, dark chocolate that is not at least 70% cacao, and chocolate that contains ingredients like soy lecithin, a food additive used as an emulsifier in many processed foods.

- Bobo's Oat Bars: (They make several varieties, such as coconut, chocolate chip, maple pecan, lemon poppyseed, and original.) They contain mostly organic ingredients but, because they contain 18-20 grams of sugar per bar, I normally eat only half a bar at a time and save the other half for another time.

- Dates or figs: While these are natural fruits, they have a higher sugar content, so I try not to eat too much of them.

- Apple with organic almond butter.

There are countless choices for dessert and snacks. It is best to choose desserts and snacks that contain few ingredients, are minimally processed, and contain a low amount of sugar. As you eat less sugar, your taste buds will adapt, and you might find that foods you once enjoyed have become too sweet for you.

Drinks

Most of the liquid that I consume is pure water, but I also drink a flavored water made by "bai". I don't drink alcohol often, but when I do, I mostly stick to red wine and an occasional dark beer.

Again, preparing meals does not have to be complicated and time-consuming. There are tons of cookbooks and websites that cater to people who want to eat healthily. Two books containing good information and recipes are, "The Guide to Healthy Eating," by David Brownstein, M.D., & Sheryl Shenefelt, C.N., and "Eat Right 4 Your Type, The Individualized Blood Type Diet Solution", by Peter J. D'Adamo and Catherine Whitney. (Note: My diet is not appropriate for everyone, as we all have different needs, and especially if you are not blood type A, as I am).

Intermittent Fasting

Just as what you eat is important, so is when you eat. Some people believe it is best to eat three meals a day, while others believe it is better to eat every few hours during the day. Our bodies were not meant to eat continuously and to digest food all day long; we need time to process and digest food. That's where intermittent fasting comes in.

There are various methods of intermittent fasting, which in its simplest form, is not eating food for a long period of time - such as 12-14 hours - on a regular basis. Our ancestors did not eat all day and evening as we do today, because food was scarcer and not as convenient and plentiful as it is today. Back then, it was often feast or famine. Studies have shown that intermittent fasting can help people lose weight, reduce blood pressure, reduce blood glucose levels, improve cholesterol and triglyceride levels, reduce inflammation, enhance muscle endurance, and improve learning and memory.[39] According to Dr. Joseph Mercola, "Training your body to burn fat for fuel and eating only during an eight-to-ten hour window creates the conditions your body needs to function optimally and to repair itself and ward off diseases effortlessly".[40]

The best way to fast intermittently is to restrict eating to certain times of the day, such as between 8 a.m. and 6 p.m., which gives you a 10-hour time frame to eat, and a 14-hour time frame to fast. Since a big part of that fasting time occurs while you are sleeping, it is not very difficult to do. You may even decide to eat breakfast a little later, or skip it altogether, to increase the fasting period. A big problem for many people is eating at night, while watching TV. "Eating at night, in particular, interferes with the body's natural day-night cycle, disrupting hormones in a way that favors weight gain."[41]

The benefits to intermittent fasting are that it:[42]

- Reduces cravings for sugar and other unhealthy foods
- Promotes human growth hormone
- Normalizes hunger levels
- Boosts your brain health
- Dramatically lowers your risk of cardiovascular disease
- Inhibits the aging process
- Helps treat or prevent cancer
- Improves gut bacteria.

If you decide to try intermittent fasting, start slowly and gradually increase the time between dinner and breakfast. If you have any medical conditions, you should discuss intermittent fasting with your doctor.

Summary

This chapter covered a lot of material on proper diet and nutrition. By now, your head might be spinning from all of this information about food, some of which you may have believed to be good for you when in fact it's actually unhealthy, and some of which you may have believed to be bad for you, when in fact it's actually good for you. Don't take my word for it, look it up for yourself. A lot of this is common sense – we all know that cake, cookies, chips, soda, and other processed junk food is not good for us, but do we understand how much damage eating these foods is doing to our bodies? We also know that we need to eat more fruits, vegetables, and other healthy foods, but do we understand that not including these foods in our diet is actually harming us? It took me years to learn this material, but hopefully, by including all this information in this book, I will save you an enormous amount of time. For those who want to learn more, I've listed several recommended books and movies at the end of Chapter 16.

CHAPTER 12:
TAKE CHARGE OF YOUR HEALTHCARE DECISIONS

"The physician must be able to tell the antecedents, know the present, and foretell the future – must mediate these things, and have two special objects in view with regard to disease, namely to do good or to do no harm."

~ Hippocrates

This is a great declaration by Hippocrates. I do believe that most physicians are in practice to help their patients improve their health. But for the most part, physicians are mainly taught how to diagnose illnesses and prescribe and utilize drugs to treat those illnesses. "This might surprise you, but medical schools don't actually train students about the importance of health or diet or nutrition. Rather, the schools place an emphasis on making a diagnosis and treating the symptoms they see with pharmaceutical drugs".[1] Dr. David Brownstein is a conventionally trained doctor who had no interest in holistic medicine early in his career. When he started seeing and treating patients with medications, Dr. Brownstein noticed that most of his patients were not getting better. It also dawned on him that he was not treating the underlying causes of his patients' illnesses, and the drugs he prescribed were only masking their symptoms. He realized he was taught little in medical school about the nature of health and how to maintain it, and he began to contemplate how he could improve his patients' health. After these realizations, Dr. Brownstein began practicing holistic medicine, and now runs a successful practice, often working with holistic dentists, pharmacists, chiropractors, and nutritionists to help his patients. According to Dr. Brownstein, holistic medicine is utilizing "a combination of conventional and alternative practices that address a patient's overall health rather than merely treating the symptoms of a particular illness".[2]

More than half of the American population takes at least one prescription drug daily, and about half of those people take four different medications.[3] In general, healthcare is very reactive when, it should be more proactive. Modern medicine tends to ignore the problem and mask the symptoms. Instead of diagnosing and treating disease, or the symptoms of disease, healthcare should emphasize the prevention of disease. Until it does, I suggest that people practice disease prevention on their own. Otherwise, it's not a matter of if people will get sick, it's a matter of when.

It is extremely important to take charge of your healthcare decisions; you must be your own health advocate. It is also especially important to find the right doctor, one who is willing to spend time with you, answer all your questions, and explain things clearly. If you are struggling with a health issue, it also pays to get a second opinion. "Studies have shown that patients who are actively engaged in their health and care experience better health outcomes. Their habits and behaviors support good health and effective treatments."[4] Consider going to a naturopathic doctor (ND) or a doctor that practices holistic medicine. Like good detectives, these types of doctors seek to find the cause of their patients' illnesses with the intention of providing a remedy to improve their health, instead of just managing disease and treating the symptoms with drugs. According to Dr. Brownstein, over the past 70 years, our food supply has seen a steady decline of vitamins and minerals, due to depleted soil.[5] "Unfortunately, you can't rely on your doctor to understand your nutritional health unless he or she has been properly trained to evaluate a patient's micronutrient levels.[6] An ND or other holistic doctor will order blood tests to identify any nutritional and hormonal deficiencies. They use the results to create a treatment program that might include dietary recommendations and vitamin and mineral supplements. This makes more sense than ignoring the cause of the problem and treating the symptoms with drugs that are foreign to the human body and may even create additional problems. Of course, there are instances when doctor-prescribed drugs can be helpful, but they should not be the long-term solution. If drugs are warranted, the GoodRx app or card might save you money on prescriptions. I work with a naturopathic doctor to help manage my own health, including vitamin and mineral deficiencies. Again, my emphasis is on prevention of disease and being proactive; I don't want to wait until I have a health problem. To find a holistic doctor near you, visit https://www.acam.org/default.aspx.

Lab Testing

In addition to any lab tests your doctor normally orders for you, you might consider having the following tested as well:

- Your hemoglobin A1C, which measures your average blood sugar over a ninety-day period. This is one of the most important medical tests to determine your present health and predict your future health.
- Your fasting blood glucose level
- Your fasting insulin levels
- Your cholesterol levels
- Your lipoprotein levels
- Your homocysteine levels
- Your vitamin D level
- Your vitamin B levels
- Your hormone levels
- Your thyroid levels (TSH, T4, T3, and thyroid antibodies)
- Your iron levels
- Other vitamin or mineral tests, as determined by your doctor

A full CardioMetabolic (CM) test covers many of these items and more. As part of my own care, I have a CM test performed every 6 months. As I mentioned, I am under the care of an ND, who is advising me on the proper types and dosages of vitamin and mineral supplements. It is especially important to work with a physician who is knowledgeable on vitamins and mineral supplements; this is not something you should do on your own. Taking the wrong types or dosages of vitamins or supplements can create an imbalance in the body and will do more harm than good. Again, I want to emphasize the importance of the prevention of disease, as opposed to hoping for the best, or waiting for disease to occur and then reacting to the problem.

In addition to working with my ND, I also see a cardiologist every so often to check my heart health. On a recent visit, I noticed a poster on the wall entitled, "Tips for Taking Your Diabetes and Cardiovascular Care Into

Your Own Hands". Under the section on cholesterol, it stated: "Taking a high-intensity statin is the single most important way to reduce cholesterol as well as your risk of heart disease and stroke". Really? Taking a pill is more important than a healthy diet and exercise? I wonder which drug company designed the poster. According to Dr. Jeffrey Perlmutter, a board-certified neurologist, the brain needs cholesterol to thrive and properly function, and when cholesterol levels are low, the brain simply doesn't work well, and individuals with low cholesterol are at much greater risk for dementia and other neurological problems.[7] There are plenty of "natural" ways to reduce cholesterol (like exercising and eating the right foods), instead of taking a high-intensity statin.

Oral Care

The medical community tends to treat each part of the body separately, with little connection among the parts, including the mouth. If you have a dental problem, you go see a dentist. Many people don't like going to the dentist, and therefore, put it off. They don't realize that problems in the mouth can greatly affect other parts of the body. Poor oral health can contribute to endocarditis, cardiovascular disease, pregnancy and childbirth complications, and pneumonia. "It is impossible to achieve your optimum health if you have poor oral hygiene."[8]

Mercury Fillings

Mercury fillings are known as amalgam, which is 50% mercury by weight. Mercury is unquestionably toxic and does not belong in the mouth. It damages the immune and endocrine systems. Several illnesses, including Alzheimer's disease, infertility, birth defects, food allergies, multiple sclerosis and other autoimmune diseases, thyroid and other hormonal problems, and cardiovascular problems, have been associated with mercury toxicity.[9] The American Dental Association (ADA) would like us to believe that amalgam fillings are safe, and that the mercury will not leach out into the body. But some studies show that mercury from amalgam fillings can be absorbed into the mouth as vapor. The amount of vapor released from amalgam fillings increases with the ingestion of hot liquids, teeth brushing, and teeth grinding. Amalgam is so toxic that dentists are not allowed to flush it down the drain and must dispose of it as hazardous material.[10] When I learned about this, I had all my amalgam fillings replaced with porcelain composites. Even though

I did not have any symptoms of mercury exposure, I did not want to take any chances. I went to a holistic dentist, who is knowledgeable about removing amalgam fillings and who follows strict procedures to make sure that the mercury exposure is minimal during the procedure. To find a holistic dentist near you, log onto: http://holisticdental.org/find-a-holistic-dentist/.

Gum Disease

Gum disease, also known as periodontitis, occurs when there is bacterial overgrowth in the periodontal tissue. It often presents as redness and swelling of the gum tissue. Gum disease can affect other parts of your body. If not treated, the bacteria from gum disease can travel through the bloodstream and affect the heart or other organs in the body, which can kill you.[11] The main way to prevent gum disease is to practice good oral hygiene. The ADA recommends that we brush our teeth at least twice a day, once in the morning and once at night before bed. Although it's a relatively simple task, many people don't brush twice a day. It is also extremely important to floss your teeth every day, to remove food stuck in between your teeth, lest it leads to gum inflammation or other issues. While a water pick is great for oral hygiene, it is not a replacement for flossing. I brush twice a day (using fluoride-free toothpaste), and floss once a day, and I have no problems with my teeth or gums. Eating a healthy diet also reduces the potential for gum and tooth disease.

Root Canals

A root canal is a procedure that is used to repair and save a decayed or infected tooth. During a root canal, the nerve and pulp of the tooth are removed, the canal is flushed with chemicals to kill any bacteria, and the tooth is cleaned out and sealed; the expectation is that the dead tooth will not later become infected. Unfortunately, even after a root canal, a dead tooth can become infected and release bacteria into the bloodstream to travel to other parts of the body. "So essentially, a root-canalled tooth is an infected mess with access to the immune system. And if it remains in the jaw, the infection level can increase requiring the immune system to work harder to contain the problem. It is well-known that an infection in one part of the body can travel to other parts. For example, a patient with a heart valve issue can develop endocarditis (inflammation of the inner layer of the heart) from dental infection. That's why patients with certain heart valve problems are often treated with antibiotics before dental procedures."[12]

I watched a good documentary on Netflix called "Root Cause," which led me to believe that, for treatment of a decayed or infected tooth, a dental implant or bridge may be a better option than a root canal.

CHAPTER 13: CANCER

"It is more important to know what sort of person has a disease than to know what sort of disease a person has."

~ Hippocrates

"The natural healing force within each of us is the greatest force in getting well."

~ Hippocrates

"Disease [is] not an entity, but a fluctuating condition of the patient's body, a battle between the substance of disease and the natural self-healing tendency of the body."

~ Hippocrates

I wanted to include a chapter on cancer, since it affects many people, including my brother, his wife, my father, my parents-in-law, my grandparents, many of my aunts and uncles, and many other people that I know or have known.

Cancer occurs when abnormal cells fail to die at the end of their life cycle; instead, they mutate and divide uncontrollably. This can result in the growth of a tumor (other than blood cancers), can impair the immune system, and can spread to other parts of the body.

The word "cancer" is one of the last things that you want to hear from your doctor's mouth. Yet, that is what my brother, Anthony, heard from his doctor in August 2010. Cancer is the second leading cause of death in the United States, just below heart disease. According to the American Cancer Society, there is about a 40 percent chance of developing cancer in a male's lifetime, and about a 38 percent chance of developing cancer in a female's lifetime; so about 4 out of every 10 people will be diagnosed with cancer in their lifetime.[1] That's pretty scary!

There are many causes of cancer, but some of the biggest risk factors are smoking, heavy alcohol consumption, excess body weight, physical inactivity, and poor nutrition. According to Dr. David Brownstein, "Many substances can disrupt the normal DNA of a cell and increase the risk of cancer. These include tobacco smoke, medical radiation, environmental toxicities, obesity, synthetic hormones, viruses, bacteria, parasites, and nutritional deficiencies."[2] According to the American Cancer Society, 87 percent of cancer cases are diagnosed in people 50 and older, so aging also appears to be a risk factor.[3] While genetics plays a role, it may not be as high as people think. "Inherited genetic mutations significantly contribute to the development of 5-10 percent of cancer cases."[4] As with other degenerative diseases, cancer often has more than one cause. As I mentioned previously, cancer is a disease that occurs in the body; it is not something that comes into our body, such as an infectious disease.

According to the Foundation for Advancement in Cancer Therapy (FACT): "... the conventional approach [to cancer treatment] believes that the tumor itself is, in effect, the disease and that cancer can be efficiently controlled by directing the therapy toward destroying the malignancy. The treatments most frequently used are radiation, chemotherapy, surgery, and hormone inhibitors, or a combination of these procedures. Thus, the major focus of this traditional approach is tumor destruction. We at FACT, on the other hand, support a concept of cancer as being a systemic malfunction which requires a biological repair. According to this concept, cancer cells are only a symptom of a dysfunction of the organism, resulting from a steady breakdown in the balance of the body chemistry. Only by restoring the balance through safe and sound biological means can the disease be truly controlled. Conjointly, we believe that if given the proper support and better lifestyle, the body's own inherent ability to repair itself could prevent cancer in the vast majority of cases".[5] "Conventional medicine is caught up in looking for a 'wonder drug' that will cure cancer all at once after diagnosis. That's the wrong approach. Instead, doctors should be training in preventive medicine so that they can minimize a patient's chance of developing cancer. Unfortunately, there is little training in prevention. The focus remains on diagnosing and prescribing drugs to treat symptoms".[6]

I wholeheartedly agree that the focus for fighting cancer should be prevention. Unfortunately, in the U.S. and many other developed nations, a lot of time and money is spent researching better diagnostic systems and better "cures" for cancer, rather than on prevention. Why is that? Because diagnosing and treating cancer is big business. In 2020, it is estimated that we will spend $158 billion on cancer care.[7] But conventional methods of cancer treatment have been mostly ineffective, as they tend to weaken the body's immune system, when, it appears that the best way to treat cancer is to improve the body's immune system. If the body's immune system is functioning well, cancer cells (which are present in most people's bodies at different times) will be destroyed by the immune system. Thus, the cancer is not allowed to progress. "Ensuring an optimally functioning immune system is important to both prevention and treatment of cancer. Remember, only your immune system can prevent cancer and only your immune system can treat cancer effectively."[8] Unfortunately, for many people, their immune system is not functioning optimally due to: a poor diet consisting of processed foods high in sugar and devoid of nutrition; a high level of toxins stored in their bodies due to a poor diet; an accumulation of poisons from the environment and from the use of noxious personal care products and cleaning products; poor elimination; high levels of stress; lack of sleep and rest; and lack of exercise.

"An anti-cancer diet (indeed, any diet) should be free of refined sugars. All cancer cells use refined sugar as a source of fuel. This was first described nearly 80 years ago by Nobel Laureate Otto Warburgh, Ph.D. He discovered that cancer cells have a different energy metabolism from normal cells. Dr. Warburgh found that cancer cells use anaerobic (without oxygen) glycolysis to produce energy. Our normal cells primarily use aerobic (with oxygen) glycolysis to produce energy. The big difference between a normal cell and a cancer cell, then, is that a cancer cell is dependent on simple sugars for their metabolic function. Thus, the best way to 'feed' a cancer cell is a diet packed with refined sugar. Dr. Warburgh also found that cancer cells produce a lot of lactic acid and live and thrive in an acidic environment. Refined sugars not only provide the necessary fuel for cancer cells, but also are very acidifying for the body. This is the perfect combination for cancer cells to thrive. White blood cells, meanwhile, are the 'policeman' of the body. They are on alert to help us fight infections and cancer. Studies have shown that ingestion of refined sugar stuns white blood cells, lowering their functionality for up to six hours."[9]

Refined sugar should be kept to a minimum, and if you are battling cancer, you should avoid it altogether.

Before cancer (or any disease) becomes a problem, a full evaluation by a holistic doctor, naturopathic doctor (ND), or other healthcare practitioner with a background in nutrition, can detect your body's nutritional deficiencies, and can correct those deficiencies before it's too late. These practitioners can also help you devise a detoxification program to remove the toxins that have been stored in the body for years. That is precisely what I am doing - working with an ND and applying the principles from this book into my own lifestyle to reduce my risk of all degenerative diseases.

One of the things I have often wondered is why some people who smoke or drink too much, or who eat an unhealthy diet and don't exercise, live a long life without disease. According to the book, "Rethinking Cancer", it has to do with "the extraordinary resilience and capacity for self-repair which Nature has bestowed upon us". The book also opines that these people may also have a strong constitution, they tend to take things in stride, and achieve a state of positive thinking and relaxation. They tend to enjoy life and are gratified by small pleasures. "A healthy mind-set enables the body to derive maximum benefit from the innate healing capacity". On the contrary, someone with a weak constitution cannot get away with the same abuses that someone with a strong constitution might get away with. Some people are blessed from birth with a strong constitution, while others are not.[10] Another consideration is quality of life. Someone who is terribly ill is more likely to make the effort to get well if they feel that their life has value and is worth living. If a cancer patient does not feel that their life has meaning and is not worth living, they probably won't survive. Optimism and hope are necessary for recovery. I know a woman who was diagnosed with stage IV ovarian cancer approximately 20 years ago. After going through the conventional treatments of surgery and chemotherapy, her doctors told her there was nothing else they could do for her. Many people at that point would have given up, but she did not. She had a great desire to live and never lost hope. She used the power of positive thinking to help heal her body. She walked through the grassy fields around her house and imagined healthy cells in her body as battalions attacking the cancer cells, and she kept focusing on the positive. She worked with Dr. Joel Fuhrman, a holistic physician in Flemington, NJ, to make some positive dietary changes, and continued to exercise her mind and body, knowing that it would take time to heal. She listened to positive messages of Deepak Chopra and others, and used other alternative sources of medicine, including acupuncture, to help heal her body. Over time, her body healed itself and her condition improved. To this day, she remains cancer-free. I find her story to be very inspirational.

I have known people who died from cancer and, in every case, they were treated with either surgery, chemotherapy, radiation treatment (also known as "cut, poison, and burn"), or some other experimental treatment. While these treatments might be effective in some cases (such as in my brother's case, as the cancer had not metastasized), in other cases, particularly more advanced cases, these treatments may not be as effective. Unfortunately, many oncologists often have no knowledge about, or interest in, utilizing diet and nutrition to heal the body. Oncologists won't acknowledge that cancer is a problem that takes years, if not decades, to develop in the body, and, likewise, that it can take time and patience to repair the body. Surgery, chemotherapy, and radiation treatments might remove or reduce the cancerous tumor, but they don't fix the underlying problem or the imbalance in the body that caused the cancer to form in the first place. In fact, chemotherapy and radiation will weaken an already weakened body, which makes it difficult for a genuine biological repair. That is why, in many cases, the cancer returns. On the other hand, a healing approach aimed at helping the whole-body repair itself will have better long-term results, especially if the individual permanently improves their diet and lifestyle. "A successful cancer therapy is one that takes into account the whole body and mind; has a clinically proven pattern of repair; uses non-toxic, non-invasive, diagnostic methods to find out where the biological break-down is and what is causing it; and then addresses the problems with an integrated repair program of biological therapy."[11]

What to Do if You Are Diagnosed With Cancer

For a cancer patient, it is important to take an active role in the healing process, not a passive role that is directed solely by his or her doctor. This means educating themselves about cancer and the various treatment options. One of the reasons I educate myself about cancer is that, if I or another family member becomes ill with cancer, I want to be aware ahead of time of the various treatment options available. It is important for the cancer patient to be aware of the different therapies for treating cancer, and to work with a doctor who will focus on the individual patient's health problems and needs. It is also important to understand that most cancer takes years, if not decades to form in the body and you should not rush to a treatment, just because your doctor pressures you to make quick decisions about your therapy.

An invaluable resource is the book, "Rethinking Cancer," by Ruth Sackman, which I highly recommend to everyone, regardless of their present health condition. I have read the book multiple times and will read it again in the future as a refresher. The book discusses many aspects of health and nutrition, as well as several non-traditional methods of cancer treatment, like "The Gerson Therapy". I also highly recommend watching the documentary, "The Gerson Miracle" (available on YouTube), which discusses this natural treatment program for cancer (I have watched the movie several times). It is better to be prepared and know your options ahead of time, instead of rushing to make hasty decisions, while facing fear, anxiety, and pressure from your doctors, family, and friends.

CHAPTER 14:
MAINTAIN A ROUTINE

Over the years, I have developed many routines in my life. I like having a routine, because once something becomes second nature, it is easier to remain consistent. Some of my routines serve the purpose of maintaining excellent health. Here are some of my daily routines:

- **Water:** Hydrating is a great way to start the day. Upon waking, I drink a glass of water, and I drink anywhere from 60-90 ounces of water during the day, depending on how active I am.

- **Meals:** Most days, I eat breakfast around 8:30-9 a.m., lunch around 12-1 p.m., and dinner around 5:30-6:30 p.m. I follow a healthy diet most of the time (described in Chapter 11), but there are times (usually when I'm dining out or on vacation), that I deviate from my diet. Regardless, I mostly try to avoid the foods that give me digestive issues.

- **Intermittent Fasting:** I normally don't eat past 7 p.m., and I won't eat again until 8:30-9 a.m., giving me 13-plus hours every day of intermittent fasting. On weekends, I often stretch the period to 15 hours.

- **Exercise:** I work out for one hour on Sunday, Tuesday, and Thursday mornings. I don't schedule anything else during this time, as working out is a top priority I am highly committed to; I very rarely miss a workout. In addition to these formal workouts, I play pickleball and tennis 2-3 times a week. In the warmer months, I also walk several times a week, and in the winter months, I jump on my mini trampoline at home, or walk, if the weather is not too cold.

- **Meditation:** I meditate 3-4 times a week, not including the times I meditate at night, when I awaken and can't quickly fall back to sleep. I intend to add even more meditation to my week.

- **Sleep and Rest:** I always aim to get 7 to 8 hours of sleep each night, and I make this a priority. Since I wake up and have trouble going back to sleep most nights, I give myself a 9-hour timeframe to get the sleep I need. I do deep breathing exercises before going to sleep each night. On weekdays, I try to get to sleep by 10:30 p.m., and on weekends by 11:30p.m.- midnight. While I lead a regularly active life, I make sure to balance it out with rest, and I make time for reading, writing, and watching TV.

- **Dental Hygiene:** I brush my teeth twice a day and floss every night. I go for regular dental checkups every 6 months.
- **Airing Out the House:** I open windows to air out my home every weekend for at least 30 minutes.
- **Reducing Toxins:** I eat an exceptionally clean diet consisting of mainly organic foods. I rarely eat GMO food products. I use personal care products that don't contain harmful ingredients. I drink filtered or bottled spring water.

Having a routine has helped me remain consistent with my diet and exercise, getting enough sleep, and managing stress, and it is something I highly recommend.

CHAPTER 15:
BALANCE YOUR LIFE

I believe that in order to live a truly fulfilling life, that life needs to be balanced with health and wellness, positive relationships, a social life, joy, spirituality, solid finances, and a sense of purpose. As I mentioned earlier, many people live a life that is out of balance, where they focus all their attention on one aspect of their life, while neglecting other aspects. A perfect example is focusing solely on health or wealth. Spending all your time building wealth might make you a financially rich person, but it might also come at the cost of your health, your relationships with your family, or even the joy of living. Figure 15-1 below is "The Circle of Life" created by The Institute for Integrative Nutrition. The Circle of Life consists of various elements of one's life. A simple exercise to go through is to assign a number, from 1-10, for each section (1 being the lowest, 10 being the highest) to determine which areas of your life are in good shape and which areas of your life need improvement.

Figure 15-1

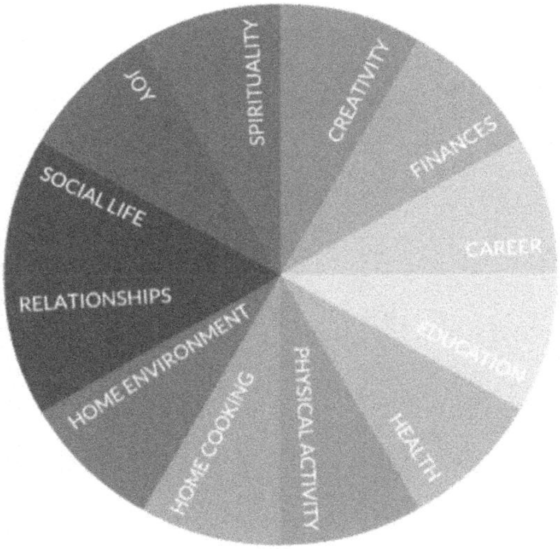

© 2005, 2015 Integrative Nutrition, Inc. | Reprinted with permission.
No further copying and/or republication is authorized.
Integrative Nutrition Inc. does not endorse the content contained in this book.

Like many people, I used to define success solely by wealth, thinking the more money you made and accumulated, and the more material things you acquired, the happier you would be. I no longer believe this fallacy. While one's financial position is important, so is your health (diet and exercise), your home environment, your relationships and social life, spirituality, creativity, career, and education. These all lead to the joy that you get out of life. As the saying goes, "stop and smell the roses". Most of us live a very busy life consumed by work and personal commitments such that we don't take the time to eat well, cook at home, exercise regularly, spend quality time with our family and friends, rest and relax, and spend time on hobbies or education. As I mentioned earlier, in certain parts of the world where people live the longest - Sardinia, Okinawa, Nicoya, Ikaria, and Loma Linda - one of the common denominators (besides diet and exercise) is having familial closeness and a close social circle.

CHAPTER 16:
FIXING OUR HEALTHCARE CRISIS

In 2018, Americans spent 3.65 trillion dollars on healthcare. That is more than the gross domestic product (GDP) of Brazil, the United Kingdom, Mexico, Spain, and Canada, and is, by far, the highest healthcare expenditure in the world. This amounts to about $11,212 per person per year.[1] Given that our spending is the highest in the world, you would think that we would have the best healthcare system in the world, but we are far from it. According to U.S. News and World Report, with respect to the best public health systems, the United States ranks #19 in the world. Here are the countries in the top 10:[2]

- Finland
- Norway
- Sweden
- Switzerland
- Canada
- Denmark
- Germany
- Netherlands
- Australia
- United Kingdom

How about life expectancies? Here is a listing of the top 20 countries with the highest life expectancies:[3]

- Monaco 89.4 years
- Japan 85.3 years
- Singapore 85.2 years
- Macau 84.6 years
- San Marino 83.3 years

- Iceland 83.1 years
- Hong Kong 82.5 years
- Andorra 82.9 years
- (tie) Guernsey 82.6 years
- (tie) Switzerland 82.6 years
- (tie) Israel 82.5 years
- (tie) South Korea 82.5 years
- (tie) Luxembourg 82.3 years
- (tie) Australia 82.3 years
- (tie) Italy 82.3 years
- Sweden 82.1 years
- (tie) Liechtenstein 81.9 years
- (tie) France 81.9 years
- (tie) Canada 81.9 years
- (tie) Norway 81.9 years

The United States ranked number 43, with an average life expectancy of 78.6 years.

So, clearly, we cannot spend our way into good health. I believe that we, as a nation, need to become better educated about health and wellness. We need to take charge of, and responsibility for, our own health, and not simply rely on a doctor to give us a pill every time we don't feel well. Our healthcare system needs to focus on the prevention of disease, instead of the diagnosis and treatment of disease. The FDA needs to be more diligent and stricter about what is allowed in our food, water, personal care products, cleaning products, and other household items we use daily. We need to vote with our wallets, and demand better food, free from the chemicals and toxic substances that are currently permitted in our food. We all need to exercise more, get more sleep, and manage stress better. It will take time before we see real change happen. My hope is that the younger generations will recognize the disaster that is our country's healthcare system and demand a change to the status quo. Only when the health of our nation improves will our healthcare costs go down.

PART I SUMMARY

Part I contains many suggestions on improving your health, including:

- Airing out your home and your office
- Reducing exposure to toxins
- Getting sufficient sunlight
- Managing stress and anxiety
- Getting sufficient sleep and rest
- Exercising
- Drinking plenty of water
- Balancing your gut bacteria
- Improving your diet
- Taking charge of your healthcare decisions
- Balancing your life.

You don't have to implement all of these at once. I didn't. I made gradual changes over time, and to this day I am still looking to make improvements. The key is to remain consistent and committed to healthy activity and behavior.

A good way to start is by implementing some of the easier changes such as replacing soda, sports drinks, fruit juices and coffee with water (remember to drink half your body weight in ounces – daily). Another easy one is to air out your house, weekly. You can also start an exercise routine; add it into your weekly schedule as a high priority activity. Once it becomes part of your routine, it becomes easier to remain consistent. It would be fairly easy to implement these three changes at the same time.

Some of the other actions will take more time and effort, but again, remember, you don't have to make all the changes at once; try adding one new change each week or each month. It took me years to learn what I know and to change my routines. This book serves as a good starting point to change your habits and routines and to improve your health.

RECOMMENDED SOURCES FOR HEALTH MANAGEMENT

Newsletters

- Dr. David Brownstein's Natural Way to Health (NewmaxHealth.com or 800-485-4350)
- Bottom Line Personal (https://bottomlineinc.com/)

Books
(These books are available on Amazon.com)

- Eat Right 4 Your Type, The Individualized Blood Type Diet Solution, Dr. Peter J. D'Adamo with Catherine Whitney
- Effortless Healing, Dr. Joseph Mercola
- Grain Brain, David Perlmutter, M.D.
- Healing Multiple Sclerosis, Ann Boroch, C.N.C.
- Rethinking Cancer, Ruth Sackman
- The Guide to Healthy Eating, David Brownstein, M.D., and Sheryl Shenefelt, C.N.
- Wheat Belly, William Davis, M.D.

Movies
(These movies might be available on Netflix or YouTube)

- Cowspiracy
- Fat, Sick, and Nearly Dead, I and II
- Fed Up
- Food Choices

- Food, Inc.
- Food Matters
- Forks Over Knives
- Hungry for Change
- In Defense of Food
- Live and Let Live
- Pet Fooled
- River of Waste
- Root Cause
- Stink
- Sugar Coated
- Supersize Me
- The C Word
- The Devil We Know
- The Gerson Miracle
- The Magic Pill
- What the Health?
- What's with Wheat?

PART II: WEALTH MANAGEMENT

INTRODUCTION

Retirement

Thinking about retirement may elicit many pleasant thoughts, such as not working or having to commute to work, waking up later, having more free time, visiting with children and grandchildren, socializing with friends, dining out, and traveling. But, in retirement, there are many challenges and risks that require a great deal of planning in advance. Typically, this is the time when you no longer receive a paycheck, you stop saving money, and you convert your hard-earned assets into an income stream to add to other forms of retirement income, such as Social Security and a pension (if you are lucky to have one). Of course, retirement looks different to each person. Some people stop working altogether, while others continue to work part-time or become volunteers. According to Pew Research, 19% of people age 65 and older are working, and this figure has been rising for the past 20 years. This working group of people is the fastest growing group in the U.S.[1]

Filling free time in retirement can be challenging for many people, especially if they worked long hours and had little time to develop interests and hobbies outside of work. Before retiring, it might be a good idea to think about what you will do with your free time, and perhaps start to cultivate hobbies and other activities. Consider your passions and interests, professional pursuits, ongoing learning, spirituality, giving back to your community, and family and friends.

Developing a Retirement Income Plan

One of the first steps to developing a retirement income plan is to take a full and accurate assessment of your assets (what you own), your liabilities (what you owe), your sources of retirement income, and your living expenses.

Your living expenses can be broken into three categories:

1. Essential or basic needs: This includes food, shelter, clothing, health care costs, taxes, etc.
2. Discretionary: This includes travel, dining out, entertainment, club memberships, etc.

3. Legacy: This is the money you may want to gift or pass on to your heirs.

Next, you'll want to "crunch" the numbers to see where you stand financially and determine if you have enough assets and income to meet your retirement income goals. At the very least, you should have enough income to cover your essential living expenses, plus a buffer for unforeseen expenses. You should also understand how much investment risk you will need to take or are willing to take, to meet these goals. Next, you should consider your investment objectives, and what you are looking to achieve. The goal of investing should not be to beat the markets; the goal should be to meet your financial objectives. A financial advisor experienced in working with retired clients and clients in the process of retiring can help you to develop a retirement plan that considers the above information.

Risks in Retirement

As previously mentioned, there are many financial risks that could arise in retirement. Here are some to consider:

- **Healthcare Spending Risk:** The risk of rapidly spending down your assets due to an accident or catastrophic illness, and not having the right healthcare coverage
- **Long-Term Care Risk:** The loss of ability to live independently, which can cause you to spend down assets to pay for your care or your spouse's care
- **The Death or Divorce of a Spouse/Partner**
- **Not Having a Proper Estate Plan**
- **Taxes in Retirement**
- **Bad Advice, Scams, Fraud, and Identity Theft**
- **Longevity Risk:** The risk of outliving your money
- **Withdrawal Risk:** The risk of taking high withdrawals that deplete your accounts
- **Sequence of Returns Risk:** The risk that withdrawals will quickly deplete your savings if there are negative market returns early in retirement

- **Investment Risk, Including:**
    - Market risk: The possibility of losing money in the securities markets
    - Investment concentration risk: The risk of having a large portion of your assets in one or a limited amount of investments
    - Interest rate risk: The risk that interest rates remain low, forcing investors to either withdraw higher amounts from their retirement savings or invest more aggressively in search of higher yields; rising interest rates can also create risk as some fixed income investments, such as bonds and preferred stocks, could decrease in value as interest rates rise.
    - Credit risk: The risk of loss from a borrower's failure to repay a loan or meet contractual obligations
    - Call risk/reinvestment risk: The risk that your investments will be called/sold prior to maturity, and you are unable to reinvest cash flows at a rate equal to that investment
    - Inflation risk: The risk that your investment income or purchasing power will be worth less in the future
- **Investment Behavior:** The risk that an investor's behavior will negatively impact their investment returns

These risks might not only affect your finances; they might also cause a lot of stress and anxiety. In the following chapters, we will discuss these risks in more detail, and suggest strategies to help mitigate these risks.

CHAPTER 1:
HEALTHCARE SPENDING RISK

When assessing the various risks in retirement, one of the first places to start is healthcare spending. The first half of this book discussed ways to improve your health. But even if you were to improve your health, because there are no guarantees in life, it is prudent to consider how healthcare costs will impact your retirement. According to the 2017 Retirement Health Care Costs Data Report, the lifetime retirement healthcare costs for an average 65-year-old couple who retired in 2017, including Medicare Parts B & D, supplemental insurance, dental insurance, deductibles, co-pays, and other out of pockets costs, total $404,253.[1] These healthcare costs are expected to increase annually by 4.22% on average, but retirees that make lifestyle changes can reduce these expenses, extend their lives, and have a higher quality of life.[2] In general, the better your health, the lower your healthcare expenses should be. Your overall health, as well as your spouse's/partner's health, should be considered when making the following retirement decisions:

- When to stop working
- When to start receiving Social Security income
- When to start receiving pension income
- When to start taking withdrawals from your qualified retirement plans and IRAs
- Annual investment portfolio withdrawal rate (example: 3% of previous year's balance)
- Investment portfolio risk
- Managing longevity risk
- Managing sequence of return risk

Understanding Medicare

Before you reach age 65, there are several important decisions you need to make about your health coverage. If you don't enroll in Medicare when you first become eligible, you might have to pay a late-enrollment penalty, and could end up with a gap in coverage (unless you have health insurance with creditable coverage, which meets a minimum set of qualifications). The initial enrollment period for Medicare is a seven-month period that:

- Begins three months before the month of your 65th birthday,
- Includes the month you turn age 65, and
- Ends three months after the month of your 65th birthday.

Part A Coverage (Hospital Coverage)

When eligible, most people should enroll in Part A coverage. Most people do not pay a premium for Part A coverage, if they, or their spouses, contributed through their paychecks for at least 40 quarters (10 years). Part A is subject to a deductible and copays. Medicare Part A covers the following:

- Inpatient hospital care
- Skilled nursing facility care
- Hospice
- Home health care
- Lab tests
- Surgery

Part B Coverage (Medical Insurance)

Deciding when to sign up for Part B is discussed on pages 150 and 151. Part B is also subject to a deductible and copays. Medicare Part B covers the following:

- Medically necessary services, including services to diagnose and treat a condition
- Preventative services, such as flu shots, or tests that can detect an illness at an early stage when treatment might be more effective
- Ambulance services

- Durable medical equipment, such as wheelchairs and crutches
- Mental health
- A second opinion before medically necessary surgery
- Limited outpatient prescription drugs

What's Not Covered by Medicare Part A and Part B

Medicare Part A and Part B coverage is subject to deductibles, co-insurance, and copays. In addition, there are certain medical expenses that are not covered by Medicare. These include:

- Long-term care
- Most dental care
- Eye exams related to prescription eyeglasses
- Dentures
- Cosmetic surgery
- Acupuncture
- Hearing aids and exams for fitting them
- Routine foot care

Part D Coverage (Prescription Drugs)

Medicare prescription drug coverage is an optional benefit. If you don't opt for Medicare drug coverage when you are first eligible, you will most likely pay a late-enrollment penalty if you join later (unless you have creditable prescription drug coverage, which meets a minimum set of qualifications). Part D covers most outpatient prescription drugs. For a list of covered prescription drugs, please visit: https://www.medicare.gov/drug-coverage-part-d/what-drug-plans-cover.

The costs for Medicare drug coverage include:

- Your premium
- The yearly deductible
- Copayments and coinsurance

- Costs in the coverage gap (known as "donut hole")
- Out of pocket costs if you get Extra Help (Extra Help is a program to help people with limited income and resources pay Medicare prescription drug program costs, including premiums, deductibles, and coinsurance.)
- Costs if you pay a late-enrollment penalty

Your actual drug plan costs will vary depending on:

- The drugs you use
- The plan you choose
- Whether your pharmacy is in your plan's network
- Whether the drugs you use are on your plan's "formulary," or list of covered drugs
- Whether you get Extra Help paying your Medicare Part D costs

Unlike most employer-sponsored group insurance, Part D does not have an out-of-pocket cap. This is an important consideration if you are taking expensive specialty drugs.

How Medicare Works with Other Insurance Coverage

If you have other health insurance coverage in addition to Medicare, "coordination of benefits" rules decide which plan pays first. The "primary" payer pays up to the limits of its coverage. The "secondary" payer pays only if there are costs that the primary payer did not cover. If you have group insurance coverage through your employer (or your spouse's employer), which insurer becomes primary and which becomes secondary is determined by the size of the employer. If the employer has 20 or more employees, then your group insurance becomes primary and Medicare is secondary. In that instance, you might not need to sign up for Part B because it is secondary, but you should still sign up for Part A, since there typically is no cost for Part A, so there is no downside. If the employer has fewer than 20 employees, the group coverage becomes secondary to Medicare, and if you don't sign up for Medicare, you will have to pay most of your medical bills out of pocket. In that instance, you should sign up for both Part A and Part B.

If you are uncertain whether your employer has 20 or more employees, ask the HR department and the health insurance carrier for clarification. If the group shrinks down to fewer than 20 employees, you should immediately sign up for Part B. In addition, if you have health insurance coverage with an employer that has 20 or more employees, then you might not need to sign up for Part D coverage, as long as the group drug coverage is considered "creditable coverage," which meets a minimum set of qualifications. If it isn't, then you should sign up for Part D drug coverage during your initial enrollment period to avoid any late penalties.

You can reject your automatic enrollment in Medicare Part B by following the instructions that are mailed to you with your Medicare enrollment packet. But after your employment or your employer-based coverage (or your spouse's coverage) ends, make sure you follow the Part B enrollment rules found on the Medicare website to avoid facing penalties.

Premiums for Medicare Coverage

The higher your income, the higher your premiums are for Part B and Part D coverage. Your premium is determined by your modified adjusted gross income (MAGI), (your adjusted gross income, plus any tax-exempt interest income reported on your federal tax return) two years prior to enrolling. You may want to speak to your tax or financial professional to see if they have any suggestions on how you can limit your gross income. If you are subject to a higher premium, known as an income-related monthly adjustment amount (IRMAA), and you have a life-changing event - work stoppage, work reduction, loss of pension income, loss of income-producing property, employer settlement payment, marriage, divorce/annulment, or death of a spouse - you may submit an SSA-44 form to Social Security to request a reduction of your IRMAA. The form can be found at https://www.ssa.gov/forms/ssa-44-ext.pdf.

Medicare enrollees may elect to have their Part B premiums automatically deducted from their Social Security benefits, or they can pay them separately. If you delay taking Social Security benefits, you must pay the Medicare premiums separately. But once you start collecting Social Security income, you should elect to have Medicare premiums deducted from your Social Security income. There are two reasons to do this: (1) convenience, and (2) if your Medicare Part B premiums are deducted from your Social Security benefits, any future increase in the Medicare premiums cannot result in a "net reduction" in Social Security benefits. In other words, any increase in Part B premiums cannot be more than the amount of your

Social Security cost-of-living adjustment. If you pay Part B separately, you don't have this protection.

For a complete breakdown of Medicare costs, including premiums, deductibles, co-insurance, and copays, visit https://www.medicare.gov/your-medicare-costs/medicare-costs-at-a-glance.

Example of Premium Breakdown

For an individual with a MAGI of $87,000 or less, and a married couple filing jointly with a MAGI of $170,000 or less, the approximate cost of Medicare Part B, Part D, and a Medigap policy in 2020 is:

   Medicare Part B: $144.60/month

  + Medicare Part D: $32.74/month

  + Medigap Policy: $157.66/month (NJ)[3]

  = Total Premiums: $335.00/month

The "Total Premiums" amount does not include deductibles, co-insurance, co-pays, dental coverage, vision coverage, or hearing coverage.

Medicare Supplement Insurance (Medigap)

On average, Medicare pays approximately 62% of an individual's health-care costs.[4] Medicare supplement insurance (Medigap) is sold through private companies, and helps pay for some of the health care costs not paid by Medicare, such as:

- Copayments
- Coinsurance
- Deductibles

In most states, Medigap policies are standardized policies that are identified by the letters A, B, C, D, F, G, K, L, M, and N. Depending on where you live, there may be up to ten different standardized Medigap policies to choose from. Each policy includes a different set of standardized benefits, and policies identified by the same letter will offer the same benefits, but premiums may vary by company. Premiums for Medigap policies can be community rated (no-age rated), issue-age rated (entry-age rated) or attained-age rated (premiums increase as you get older). Medigap policies have a separate six-month open enrollment period, which starts the month you turn 65, or when you enroll in Medicare if you are over 65. If you wait until the open enrollment period has ended, you must go through medical underwriting, and might have to pay more for the coverage.

Part C Coverage (Medicare Advantage)

About one-third of Medicare beneficiaries enroll in all-inclusive private health plans, known as Medicare Advantage Plans, which offer lower overall costs and often include additional benefits, in exchange for utilizing a network of health care providers. Part C lets you choose coverage through these private health plans instead of original Medicare coverage. Medicare Advantage Plans contract with the federal government and include HMOs and PPOs. "Medicare Advantage Plans must offer, at minimum, the same benefits as Original Medicare (those covered under Parts A and B) but can do so with different rules, costs, and coverage restrictions."[5] Medicare Advantage typically includes a regional network of physicians, so if you intend to go to doctors out of the area or who aren't included in the network, you will have to pay out of pocket. These plans may or may not include prescription drug coverage.

Choosing the right coverage will help you make the most of your Medicare benefits while managing your healthcare costs. For the most complete and comprehensive information on Medicare, please visit https://www.medicare.gov/ and https://www.medicareinteractive.org/. You may also want to speak to an insurance agent who is knowledgeable in this field.

Other Health Insurance Options

What if you or your spouse retire or terminate employment before age 65 and you don't have coverage; what are your health insurance options?

1. You could enroll in COBRA (Consolidated Omnibus Budget Reconciliation Act), which is temporary health insurance for people who lost or left their jobs, which enables them to avoid a gap in health insurance coverage. If you and your family are covered under a group health insurance plan that is eligible for COBRA coverage, your spouse and children would be covered under COBRA if:

- You die
- You get divorced
- You switch to Medicare coverage
- Your child turns age 26 and can no longer stay on your group health insurance plan

Please keep in mind that, with COBRA coverage, you are paying the full cost of the health insurance (plus a 2% administrative fee), which can be very expensive, especially since there is no longer an employer contribution (which often covers 70-80% of insurance premiums). The average cost for family health insurance is $20,576, although on average, employees with group health insurance through work pay $6,015.[6] Once you lose group health insurance coverage, you have 60 days to enroll in COBRA continuation coverage. COBRA coverage is meant to be temporary, and normally lasts up to 18 months from the time of enrollment. Under certain circumstances, you may extend benefits up to 36 months.

2. You could buy an individual health insurance plan through the health insurance marketplace. Plans vary by state. Different plans have different coverage options, so make sure you understand what is and isn't covered, and what your out-of-pocket costs are with each plan. You might also consider a high-deductible health insurance plan paired with a health savings account (HSA), which allows you to make pre-tax contributions to an account that can be used to pay out-of-pocket expenses. The health savings account can be used to cover current medical expenses or can be deferred to cover future medical expenses in retirement. Also, if you would like to stick with your existing doctors, find out which networks they participate in, and choose a plan within that network. Depending on your income, you might qualify for a premium tax credit, which can help to reduce your monthly premiums. Open enrollment for individual health insurance runs from November 1 through December 15. If your employment is terminated during the year and you lose group coverage, you may enroll in individual health insurance at that time.

To get an estimate for the cost of individual health insurance coverage and to see if you are eligible for a premium tax credit, visit https://www.kff.org/interactive/subsidy-calculator/.

CHAPTER 2: LONG-TERM CARE RISK

Understanding Long-Term Care

While addressing healthcare spending risk, another wealth-management risk in retirement is suffering from an accident or a chronic illness that causes you to spend down assets to pay for long-term care. Although health insurance might cover most, if not all of the initial medical costs, long-term care goes beyond medical care. Long-term care includes all the assistance one would need if they suffered a chronic illness or disability that left them unable to care for themselves for an extended period of time. This includes assistance with, or supervision of, the following activities of daily living (ADLs):

- Eating
- Bathing
- Dressing
- Toileting
- Transferring: the ability to move from one place to another, for example from a bed to a chair
- Continence: the ability to control bowel and bladder movements

In addition to assistance with ADLs, long-term care can also come into play for instrumental activities of daily living (IADLs), which include the following[1]:

- Companionship and mental support
- Transportation and shopping
- Preparing meals
- Managing a person's household
- Managing and taking medications

- Communicating with others
- Managing finances

Long-term care might also be needed if you suffer a severe cognitive impairment, such as dementia or Alzheimer's. Although you might never need long-term care, about 19 percent of Americans aged 65 and older experience some degree of chronic physical impairment and require long-term care. Among those age 85 or older, which is the fastest growing segment of our population, the number of those needing long-term care increases to about 55 percent. Statistics show that 22 percent of those age 85 and older live in a nursing home. In the year 2020, twelve million older Americans are expected to need long-term care. "A study by the U.S. Department of Health and Human Services indicates that people age 65 face at least a 40 percent lifetime risk of entering a nursing home sometime during their lifetime. About 10 percent will stay there five years or longer." Since women generally outlive men, they face a 50 percent greater likelihood than men of entering a nursing home after age 65.[2]

Cost of Care

Below are some national average costs for long-term care in the U.S. in 2019[3]:

- A private room in a nursing home: $8,517/month ($102,204/year)
- Semi-private room in a nursing home: $7,513/month ($90,156/year)
- An assisted-living facility: $4,051/month ($48,612/year)
- Home health aide: $4,385/month ($52,620/year)
- Homemaker services: $4,290/month ($51,480/year)
- Adult day health care center: $1,625/month ($19,500/year)

This is merely the national average; in some states, such as New Jersey and New York, the costs can be much higher.

With the help of your family and your financial advisor, you can create a plan of care, which should consider the following:

- Who do you want to care for you? This could be your spouse, your children, or a qualified professional. You should also consider how having a family member care for you would affect your family members' lives. Also, proximity to family is an important consideration as to whom should care for you.
- Where would you like to receive the care? This could be your home or a family member's home, an assisted-living facility, a community center, or a nursing home.
- How will you pay for your care? Do you have enough assets and income to pay for care? How will this financially impact your spouse/partner?

Options for Paying for Care

- **Healthcare and Medicare Insurance:** Health insurance offers only short-term or limited coverage for skilled and rehabilitative services. It does not cover ongoing care. If certain requirements are met, Medicare might cover a portion of the first 100 days of care received at a nursing facility.
- **Medicaid:** Medicaid is a government program that helps individuals with limited income pay for medical care. To qualify for Medicaid, you are forced to spend down most of your assets before coverage will begin.
- **Family:** Although family members could assume the responsibility of providing long-term care, or help pay for the costs, this might put emotional and financial stress on those family members.
- **Self-Insure:** If you have considerable assets, you might be able to self-insure by setting aside assets that could be used to pay for care, if needed.
- **Long-Term Care (LTC) Insurance:** These insurance policies might offer coverage for home healthcare and personal care services, respite care, adult day care, assisted living, nursing home care, hospice care, and other care. The type of coverage will vary by policy. In order to qualify for long-term care benefits under these policies, a licensed healthcare professional must certify that you are chronically ill and unable to perform, for a period of at least

90 days, two activities of daily living (ADLs) - eating, bathing, dressing, toileting, transferring, and continence, or that you have a severe cognitive impairment, such as dementia or Alzheimer's. Distributions from LTC insurance policies are normally tax-free for qualified long-term care expenses. Some policies reimburse for the actual qualified long-term care expenses, while others pay an indemnity benefit, regardless of the long-term care expenses incurred. If the policy offers an optional cost-of-living adjustment benefit (COLA), it might be worth considering, so that benefits can potentially keep pace with inflation. As with any insurance policy, it is best to buy a policy from a highly rated insurance company.

Different Types of Long-Term Care Policies

- **Traditional Long-Term Care Insurance:** This type of policy offers stand-alone coverage that provides flexibility in plan design and allows the policyowner to pay manageable premiums over their lifetime. Good health and partner/spousal discounts can help reduce the premiums. Premiums for this type of policy can increase and are not guaranteed to remain level. Premiums might be tax-deductible, check with your tax advisor. This type of policy is attractive to someone who wants to pay the premiums over the course of their lifetime.

- **Life Insurance with a Long-Term Care Rider:** This type of policy is permanent life insurance with an optional rider to help pay for the costs of long-term care. An LTC rider allows the policyowner to use a percentage of their death benefit to pay for long-term care. If the insured does not have an LTC claim, the full death benefit is paid income tax-free to the beneficiaries. If there is an LTC claim, it reduces the death benefit dollar for dollar. Any remaining death benefit is paid income tax-free. Premiums might be guaranteed to never increase, depending on the type of life insurance policy. This type of policy may be attractive to someone who primarily wants life insurance protection, but also wants to have some form of long-term insurance coverage.

- **Hybrid Life/Long-Term Care Insurance:** This type of policy offers life insurance with an LTC rider. If the insured does not have an LTC claim, the full death benefit is paid income tax-free to the beneficiaries. If there is an LTC claim, it reduces the death benefit dollar for dollar. Any remaining death benefit is paid income tax-free. This type of policy builds cash value and might include a full or partial return-of-premium feature, should the policyowner surrender the policy. It offers various premium payment options, including a single lump sum payment option, a 5-pay option, a 10-pay option, or a lifetime pay option. Premiums and benefits are typically guaranteed to not change. Good health and partner/spousal discounts can help reduce the premiums. The underwriting is normally a simplified process. This type of policy is especially attractive for someone who has a lump sum of money that they wish to allocate for LTC coverage, or for someone who prefers to pay premiums over a short period of time. It is also attractive to individuals who want a death benefit paid out in the event they don't need long-term care.

- **Hybrid Annuities/Long-Term Care Insurance:** Some insurance companies offer an annuity with a combined long-term care benefit rider. These annuities may be a fixed annuity, an index annuity, or a variable annuity. As the annuity account value grows, so does the amount available for long-term care expenses. Premiums are typically funded with a lump sum payment. The underwriting is normally a simplified process. This is the easiest form of LTC insurance to qualify for medically; so, for someone with significant health issues, it might be their only option for long-term care insurance. These policies are attractive to someone who wants to earn interest on their money, while being able to use it to pay for long-term care.

For more information, please visit: https://www.naic.org/documents/prod_serv_consumer_ltc_lp.pdf, or speak to a financial advisor or insurance agent. By planning ahead, you can be prepared in the event you or your spouse/partner require long-term care.

CHAPTER 3:
THE DEATH OR DIVORCE OF A SPOUSE/PARTNER

In addition to the emotional toll, the death or divorce of a spouse/partner poses many problems in retirement. First, let's discuss the death of a spouse/partner.

Part I: The Death of a Spouse/Partner

After the death of a spouse or partner, the survivor goes through a series of emotions. During this often-difficult time, friends and family can provide emotional support, and support groups, specifically those designed for grieving widows/widowers, can also be extremely helpful. In addition to the emotional toll, there is also the financial aspect of dealing with the death of the loved one. This can be an overwhelming task for the surviving spouse or partner, especially if they were not involved in the day-to-day finances of the couple. Widows are one of the fastest growing segments of the U.S. population. Over one million women are widowed in the U.S. every year; the number of widows in the U.S. is fast-approaching 13 million. In addition, 80% of women die single, while 80% of men die married. The average age of the onset of widowhood is 59.[1] Only about 8% of widows aged 55-64 remarry; by age 65, only about 2% of widows remarry (a widower typically remarries within 2-3 years of his wife's death).[2] Also of note, "A recent UBS survey found that 54% of U.S. women said their spouse takes the lead in handling the family's finances beyond paying bills. These women did not participate in long-term financial planning, investing or health-care decisions."[3] If the surviving spouse never handled the finances, suddenly having to do so can be a daunting task, leaving the widow or widower feeling less secure about financial matters. A financial advisor can be a valuable resource.

There are many financial considerations to be aware of after the death of a spouse or partner. Some of these items will be discussed next, including Social Security survivor benefits, pensions, annuities, and life insurance.

Social Security Survivor Benefits

Surviving Spouse

- Under certain circumstances, a one-time death payment of $255 will be paid to the surviving spouse, or to a child who is eligible for benefits.
- A surviving spouse and children might be eligible for the late spouse's Social Security benefits.
- Reduced benefits can be paid as early as age 60, or full benefits at full retirement age or older. If widows or widowers qualify for benefits on their own record, they may switch to their own retirement benefits as early as age 62.
- If the surviving spouse opts to receive their late spouse's higher Social Security benefits, they will lose their own benefits. If their own benefits are higher, they will lose their late spouse's benefits. So, in either case, there will be a loss of income since the surviving spouse cannot collect both spouses' Social Security benefits.
- Benefits could be paid as early as age 50 if the surviving spouse is disabled, and the disability started before or within 7 years of the deceased spouse's death.
- Benefits could be paid at any age, if the surviving spouse has not remarried and is taking care of the deceased's child who is under age 16 or disabled.

Children

- Unmarried children younger than 18 (or up to age 19 if attending elementary or secondary school full time) may be eligible to receive Social Security benefits when a parent dies.
- Children who are disabled before age 22 and remain disabled, can collect Social Security benefits at any age. In addition to biological children, stepchildren, grandchildren, step-grandchildren or adopted children, may also receive benefits under certain circumstances.

Parents

- Biological parents, stepparents, and adoptive parents may be eligible for benefits.

Amount of Social Security Survivor Benefits

How much the family receives in benefits depends on the deceased individual's average lifetime earnings. For more information on Social Security survivorship benefits, please visit: https://www.ssa.gov/planners/survivors/onyourown.html.

Pensions

Depending on the deceased individual's pension plan, there may be a survivor income. The following are different pension payout options that may be offered by the pension:

- **Single Life Payment:** This option provides guaranteed income for the life of the pensioner, but benefits end upon his or her death. This option provides the highest pension income, but there are no survivorship benefits.

- **Joint and Survivor Payment:** This option provides a reduced guaranteed income for the life of the pensioner but, upon his or her death, pension benefits continue to be paid to the surviving spouse. These benefits might equal 100%, 75% or 50% of the initial pension benefit amount, depending on the survivorship option chosen. Please keep in mind that the higher the survivorship benefit chosen, the lower the initial pension amount.

- **Period Certain Payment:** Some pension plans offer this option, which pays guaranteed income for a defined period of time. These benefits might not last for the pensioner's lifetime, but will continue for the period chosen, regardless of whether the pensioner or surviving spouse is alive.

- **Lump Sum Payment:** Some pensions plans offer the option to receive a lump sum payment, which can be received as income, or rolled over into an IRA to continue tax deferral.

If your late spouse was receiving pension income, and you are not sure if there are any survivorship benefits, you should contact the company providing the pension, the plan administrator, or your late spouse's employer. Military pensions normally end at death of the pension holder, but there is a form of insurance called a Survivor Benefit Plan (SBP) that issues a monthly payment to the surviving spouse and/or children. A surviving military spouse should check to see whether the late spouse had an SBP. Qualified surviving spouses, ex-spouses who never remarried, and unmarried dependent children of wartime veterans might also be eligible for benefits under a VA Survivor's Pension.[4]

Annuities

An annuity is an insurance policy in which you pay a set amount of money, at once or over a period of time, in exchange for a stream of income or a lump-sum payment in the future. It is essentially a contracted investment policy with an insurance company. The two phases of an annuity are:

1. **The Accumulation or Deferral Phase:** During this phase, funds grow in value as interest is credited to the annuity. The interest may be fixed or variable. (Annuity earnings will be discussed in greater detail in Chapter 12). If the annuity owner dies during this phase, the beneficiaries listed on the policy will normally have the following options when receiving the annuity's death benefit:

    - Lump sum distribution: Beneficiaries can withdraw the funds in a lump sum.

    - Five-year rule: Beneficiaries can withdraw funds during a five-year period or withdraw the entire amount in the fifth year.

    - Non-qualified stretch: Some annuities allow the beneficiaries to receive payments that could be stretched over their life expectancies.

    - Lifetime income: If the annuity included a joint guaranteed income benefit rider or joint lifetime income rider, lifetime income would be paid to the spousal beneficiary.

    - Annuitization: Provides a guaranteed income like a pension.

    - Spousal ownership change: Many annuities permit a surviving spouse to change the annuity contract into his/her name. The surviving spouse can continue to defer income taxes, take distributions, and change the beneficiaries of the annuity.

Please note that for qualified annuities (made with pre-tax contributions), if a non-spouse inherits the annuity, under the current tax law, they must withdraw all the money from the annuity within ten years of the annuity owner's death.

2. **The Annuitization or Distribution Phase:** During this phase, the owner begins to receive payments from the annuity. If the annuity owner dies while distributions are being paid, the beneficiaries might receive payments, depending on how distributions are structured in the annuity. Annuitization survivorship benefits are paid similarly to how a pension is paid, as previously described. Annuitization payout options include single life option, joint and survivor option, or period certain option. Fortunately, less than 5 percent of all annuities are annuitized, so it is less likely that the annuity was annuitized with a single life option, leaving the surviving spouse with no annuity benefit.[5] But if an annuity is annuitized with a single life annuitization option and without an installment refund option or cash refund option (described in Chapter 12), at the death of the owner, there would be no survivorship benefits. If an annuity is not annuitized and includes a joint income rider that provides guaranteed lifetime payments to both spouses, payments would continue to be paid to the surviving spouse.

Life Insurance

Life insurance can take on many forms, including individual and group life insurance, mortgage insurance, credit life insurance, accidental death and dismemberment insurance, credit card insurance, and travel insurance. Typically, death benefits are paid income-tax free in a lump sum. There are often other payment options available as well, such as an installment-payout option (paid out over a series of payments) or an annuitization option, described earlier. Death benefits are usually paid out within 30 to 60 days of a claim. However, if the insured dies within two years after a policy is issued, the claims process could take longer because of a policy's contestability period, during which the company is allowed to investigate the original insurance application to ensure that no fraud was committed. Also, a homicide could delay a payout, to rule out the beneficiary as a suspect. Most policies also have a suicide clause in place for the first two years of the policy. Thus, if the insured dies of a self-inflicted injury during the first two years of the policy, the insurance company will likely deny the claim. The suicide provision is intended to prevent an insured from buying a policy and then immediately taking their own life. Some policies offer an accelerated death benefit, which allows a policyholder to draw against the face value of the policy in the event of a terminal, chronic, or critical illness. If an accelerated death benefit is taken prior to the death of the insured, that amount is subtracted from the death benefit upon the insured's death. Also, if the policy has a cash-value component, and funds are withdrawn or borrowed during the life of the insured, the amount withdrawn or borrowed reduces the death benefit dollar for dollar.

Below is a checklist of some of the items to address after the death of a spouse/partner.

Checklist of Items to Address After the Death of a Spouse/Partner

(Immediately After Death)

- [ ] Obtain copies of the death certificate since it will be needed to file claims for benefits. A death certificate can be obtained from the funeral home, or the county or state vital records office where the death occurred. Locate estate-planning documents, such as the will and trusts, and other relevant documents, such as deeds and titles; the deceased's attorney should have copies of any estate-planning documents. Also, locate the marriage certificate, birth or adoption certificates of surviving children, and military discharge papers; these, too, might be needed to apply for benefits. These documents are likely stored in a safe, a safe-deposit box, or other secure place.

- [ ] File the will with the appropriate probate court. If you are working with an attorney, they will do this for you. If the deceased owned real estate out of state, file ancillary probate in that state as well. If there is no will, contact the probate court for instructions, or contact a probate attorney for assistance.

- [ ] Make a list of all assets and liabilities. Put safeguards in place to protect any property. Make sure all bills continue to be paid while the estate is being settled.

☐ Report the death to Social Security. You can call 1-800-772-1213, or your local SS office. The funeral home might also report the death to Social Security. Do not cash any of the deceased's outstanding Social Security checks received during the month the individual died or later; you might have to return some of the payments. For funds received by direct deposit, contact the bank or other financial institution, and request that any funds received during the month of death or later be returned to Social Security. Surviving spouses and other family members may be eligible for a lump-sum death benefit and/or a survivor's benefit. For more information, please visit https://www.ssa.gov/.

☐ Contact the deceased's workplace: Collect any salary, vacation, or sick pay owed to your loved one, and be sure to ask about continuing health insurance coverage and potential survivor's benefits for a spouse or children. Get information on any group life insurance and accidental death benefits (if the death was an accident). Unions and professional organizations might also offer death benefits. Get information on all retirement and pension plans. If the death was work-related, you might be entitled to an additional death benefit or worker's compensation benefits.

☐ Contact previous employers about retirement and pension plans and contact any IRA custodians or trustees. Review designated beneficiaries and post-death distribution options.

☐ Locate life insurance policies, which might include individual and group life insurance, mortgage insurance, credit life insurance, accidental death and dismemberment, credit card insurance, travel insurance, and annuities. Contact all insurance companies to notify them of the death.

☐ Evaluate your health insurance coverage. If you (and dependent children) were covered under your late spouse's employer group health insurance plan, and you are too young to qualify for Medicare, and you are employed, you can obtain coverage through your own employer's group plan, if offered. If a plan is not offered by your employer, or you are not employed, you might be eligible for continued health insurance coverage under your late spouse's plan through COBRA, which allows for continued coverage for up to 36 months after the death of a spouse (but you will have to pay the premiums previously paid by the deceased's employer). Another option is to buy an individual health insurance policy. Depending on your income, you might qualify for a premium tax credit.

- [ ] Contact all credit card companies to notify them of the death. Cancel all cards unless you are named on the account and wish to retain the card.

- [ ] Locate passwords to all accounts. Look for accounts that don't mail printed statements. Also look for digital accounts, including: PayPal and cryptocurrency accounts; websites; domain names; digital storage accounts, such as photos, videos, music, movies, e-books; prepaid accounts; frequent flier and other rewards accounts; social media; and email accounts.

- [ ] Re-title jointly held assets, such as bank accounts, automobiles, brokerage accounts, and real estate holdings.

- [ ] If the deceased owned, controlled, or was a principal in a business, check to see if there are any buy-sell agreements under which his or her interest must be sold. Buy-sell agreements are often funded with life insurance.

- [ ] Notify the deceased's creditors by mail and by placing a notice in the newspaper. Claims by creditors must be made within the statute of limitations, which varies from state to state (30 days from actual notice is common). Insist upon proof of all claims.

- [ ] Assure the estate is distributed to the beneficiaries. The executor of the will is normally responsible for settling the estate.

- [ ] File deceased's income tax returns and determine whether estate tax and/or inheritance tax returns must be filed. A federal estate tax return may need to be filed within 9 months of death; state laws vary. Federal and state income taxes are due for the year of death on the normal filing date unless an extension is requested. If there are trusts, separate income tax returns may need to be filed. Please seek the advice of a tax professional to help resolve these issues.

(Within 3-6 months after death - or sooner, if possible)

- [ ] Go through a cash-flow analysis to determine your income and expenses. Determine how being a widow/widower will change your tax filing status and income tax deductions.

☐ Review your short-term and long-term finances. If you (and/or your late spouse) are working with a financial advisor, meet with the advisor to discuss your financial goals and changes to your situation, and consider doing a new financial plan, even if there is a cost. If you do not have a financial advisor, or are not comfortable working with your present advisor, ask for a trusted referral from your friends and family, or from an accountant or attorney.

☐ Update or create your will, power of attorney, living will, and trusts with an estate attorney.

☐ Update the beneficiary designations on retirement accounts, IRAs, and annuities.

☐ Set up a TOD (Transfer on Death) on non-retirement investment accounts, and a POD (Payable on Death) on bank accounts. For more control, consider setting up a trust.

☐ Re-evaluate your insurance needs, including life, disability (if working), and long-term care. Update beneficiary designations on all insurance policies on which the deceased was named as beneficiary.

Part II: Divorce

The rate of divorce among Americans 50 and older has more than doubled since 1990.[6] Like losing a spouse to death, there is an emotional aspect to dealing with divorce, especially if the marriage was long-lasting, and children are involved. A divorce can also have a devastating financial impact on pre-retirees and retirees. Upon divorce, assets and income are typically divided between spouses, leaving each spouse in worse financial shape than when they were a couple. Dividing marital assets can be a difficult task for divorcing couples. Assets to be divided might include a home and other real estate holdings, vehicles, financial assets, retirement accounts, businesses, and personal items. Since state laws vary, it's important to understand your state's laws with respect to dividing marital property. For example, in states with "community property" laws, spouses retain ownership of anything they owned before the marriage, including an inheritance, but assets acquired during a marriage are owned equally. Community property states include Arizona, California, Idaho, Louisiana, Nevada, New Mexico, Texas, Washington, and Wisconsin. All other states have "equitable distribution" laws. Under these laws, "equitable distribution" does not mean "equal division," it means "fair division." Thus, the marital property is divided between the spouses in a fair and equitable manner. Instead of splitting assets between spouses 50/50, the future financial situation of each spouse is considered by the court making the equitable distribution decision.

Assets

Prior to the dividing of assets, the first step is to make a list of all individually owned and jointly owned assets, including:

- Your primary residence, vacation homes, investment properties, land, and other real estate holdings
- All vehicles, recreational vehicles, and boats
- Bank and credit union accounts
- Investment accounts
- IRAs and other qualified retirement accounts (plans that meet ERISA guidelines)
- Non-qualified retirement accounts (plans that don't meet ERISA guidelines)
- Stock options and employee stock ownership plans (ESOP)
- Annuities
- Life insurance policies
- Business interests
- Furniture, art, antiques, jewelry, family heirlooms, and other personal property

Disputes can occur over the distribution of property when spouses are not in agreement. Divorce mediators or divorce attorneys can be hired to solve this problem, but at a cost. Many divorces are settled without going through trial, using a property division agreement. If the ex-spouses can work together in dividing assets, the process will be smoother and less expensive. Typically, the most difficult assets to divide between spouses are retirement accounts and family-owned businesses. Retirement assets are often split up using a Qualified Domestic Relations Order (QDRO) document. Dividing a business can be complicated, because the value of the business, as well as the present and future profits, must be determined first, and that is often a difficult task. Accountants and business valuation companies can help.

Liabilities

In addition to a list of all assets, make a list of all liabilities (debts), including:

- Mortgages
- Home equity loans and lines of credit
- Auto and other vehicle loans
- Credit card debt
- Student loans
- Outstanding medical bills
- Other debt

Income

Next, make a list of all income sources, including:

- Earned income
- Unearned income from investments and properties
- Social Security
- Other government benefits
- Pension income
- Annuity income
- Business income
- Other income

A good reference point for determining income is your most recent tax return.

Social Security Benefits

Social Security benefits must be considered, especially if one spouse earned significantly more than the other. Even after divorce, you are entitled to receive part of your ex-spouse's Social Security benefits if:

1. Your marriage lasted 10 years,
2. You are 62 or older,
3. You are unmarried,
4. Your ex-spouse is entitled to receive Social Security retirement or disability benefits,

   AND

5. The Social Security benefit based on your work record is less than that based on your ex-spouse's record. (Keep in mind that, if your retirement benefit is higher than your ex-spouse's benefit, they may be entitled to part of your benefits after divorce).

Other Factors to Keep in Mind with Social Security

- If you don't remarry, you are entitled to receive half of your ex-spouse's Social Security benefits at his/her normal retirement age.

- You can collect on your ex-spouse's benefits, even if your ex-spouse delays filing for benefits, but the benefits would be permanently reduced if you begin taking them before your full retirement age. You would continue to receive these benefits even if your spouse remarries. But if you remarry, you generally cannot collect benefits on your ex-spouse's record unless your subsequent marriage ended by death, divorce, or annulment prior to you filing for your ex-spouse's benefits.

- If you start receiving benefits at your full retirement age, your benefit, as a divorced spouse, is equal to one-half of your ex-spouse's full retirement benefits amount (or disability benefits).

- If your ex-spouse has not applied for retirement benefits but qualifies for them, you can receive benefits on the ex-spouse's record if you have been divorced for at least two years.

- If you are eligible for retirement benefits on your own record and on your ex-spouse's record, the Social Security Administration will pay your retirement benefits first. If the benefit on your ex-spouse's record is higher, you will receive the additional amount based on your ex-spouse's record, giving you a combination of benefits equal to that higher amount.

- If you were born before January 2, 1954, and have already reached your full retirement age, you may choose to receive only your ex-spouse's benefit, and delay receiving your retirement benefit until a later date. If you were born on January 2, 1954 or later, you do not have this option; if you file for benefits, you will be filing for all personal and spousal benefits.

- The amount of benefits you receive does not affect the amount of benefits received by your ex-spouse or his/her current spouse.

Social Security Benefits Upon the Death of a Divorced Spouse

Upon the death of a divorced spouse, you may be eligible to receive the deceased's Social Security benefits.

- A surviving divorced spouse may qualify for the same benefits as a widow or widower (see Chapter 3, Part I), if they were married to the deceased for 10 years or more. If the surviving divorced spouse qualifies for retirement benefits on their own record, they may switch to their own Social Security retirement benefit as early as age 62.

- The payment of the deceased's benefits to a surviving divorced spouse does not affect the benefit amounts received by other survivors of the deceased.

- If the surviving divorced spouse remarries after reaching age 60, (age 50 if disabled), the remarriage does not affect their eligibility for survivor's benefits.

- A surviving divorced spouse does not have to meet the length-of-marriage rule to receive the deceased's benefits if they are caring for the deceased's child, is under age 60, or is disabled. The child must be a biological or legally adopted child. The payment of these benefits might affect the amount of benefits other survivors will receive on the deceased's earnings record.

For more information, please visit: https://www.ssa.gov/benefits/retirement/planner/applying7.html and https://www.legalzoom.com/articles/dividing-assets-what-to-do-in-a-divorce. It may also be helpful to speak to a divorce attorney or mediator. Handling finances on your own can be an overwhelming task, especially if you were not involved in the marriage's day-to-day finances. A financial advisor can be a valuable resource for a divorcee.

Below, is a checklist of some of the items to address after a divorce.

Checklist of Items to Address After a Divorce is Settled

- ☐ Make a list of your assets and liabilities.
- ☐ Go through a cash flow analysis to determine your income and expenses. Consider how divorce will change your tax filing status and deductions. (Alimony was once tax deductible for the payor, and taxable to the recipient, but that is no longer the case).
- ☐ Review your short-term and long-term finances. If you have a financial advisor, meet with the advisor to discuss your financial goals and changes, and consider having a financial plan drafted, even if there is a cost. If you do not have a financial advisor, or are not comfortable working with your present advisor, ask for a referral from your friends and family or accountant or attorney.
- ☐ Evaluate your health insurance coverage. If you were covered under your ex-spouse's employer group health insurance coverage, and you are too young to qualify for Medicare, and you are employed, you can obtain coverage through your own employer's group plan, if such a plan is offered. If a plan is not offered by your employer, or you are not employed, you might be eligible for continued health insurance coverage under your ex-spouse's benefits through COBRA, which allows for continued coverage for up to 36 months after a divorce. Another option is to buy an individual health insurance policy. Depending on your income, you might qualify for a premium tax credit.
- ☐ Update your will, power of attorney, living will, and trusts with an estate attorney.
- ☐ Update the beneficiary designations on retirement accounts, IRAs,

and annuities.

- [ ] Set up a TOD (Transfer on Death) on non-retirement investment accounts, and a POD (Payable on Death) on bank accounts. For more control, consider setting up a trust.

- [ ] Re-title jointly held assets, such as bank accounts, automobiles, stocks and bonds, and real estate holdings.

- [ ] Re-evaluate your insurance needs, including life, disability (if working), and long-term care. Update beneficiary designations on all insurance policies. Note: the divorce agreement could require that an ex-spouse be listed as the primary beneficiary on a life insurance policy, or, alternatively, could require the purchase of additional life insurance.

- [ ] Contact all credit card companies and cancel or change joint credit cards.

- [ ] Change passwords and PIN numbers on all personally owned accounts, including accounts that don't mail printed statements. Update your personal digital accounts, including: PayPal and cryptocurrency accounts; websites; domain names; digital storage accounts, such as photos, videos, music, movies, and e-books; prepaid accounts; frequent flier and other rewards accounts; social media; and email accounts.

Additional Points to Consider After the Death or Divorce of a Spouse

Regardless of how someone becomes single, here are some additional things to consider[7]:

- Don't rush into making any big decisions, such as moving or buying a house.
- Allow time to adjust.
- Beware of con artists and other unscrupulous people.
- Becoming single may mean having to step out of your comfort zone.
- Build new friendships that fit your new life.

- Join support groups for the newly divorced or widowed. You will meet people going through a similar experience.
- Join local clubs that fit your interests. You will meet like-minded people.
- Use your new single status to focus on your health, diet, and exercise.

CHAPTER 4:
NOT HAVING A PROPER ESTATE PLAN

Many people think they don't need an estate plan because they don't have a large estate. But consider this - your estate includes *everything* you own, such as:

- Your primary residence, vacation homes, investment properties, land, and other real estate holdings
- All vehicles, recreational vehicles, and boats
- Checking, savings accounts, CDs, and other cash instruments
- Investment accounts
- IRAs and qualified retirement accounts (plans that meet ERISA guidelines)
- Non-qualified retirement accounts (plans that don't meet ERISA guidelines)
- Stock options and employee stock ownership plans (ESOP)
- Annuities
- Life insurance
- Business interests
- Furniture, art, antiques, jewelry, family heirlooms, and other personal property

Even if you haven't accumulated a great deal of *wealth*, you should still have an estate plan in place to deal with the disbursement of the many categories of assets that make up your estate. You may want to choose how your possessions are bestowed to your loved ones, or to charities, after you have passed on. Traditional estate planning focuses primarily on what you own at your death, to whom you want to leave your possessions, and when you want the assets distributed, all while paying the least amount in taxes, legal fees, and court costs. While financial assets are important when considering your estate plan, your legacy - your family's values, history, traditions, and memories - should also be considered. A proper estate plan starts with a Last Will and Testament.

Last Will and Testament

A valid Last Will and Testament describes how your assets are to be distributed at your death. An executor, named by you in the will, has the responsibility to distribute your estate according to your wishes, as described in the will. Any assets titled in your name, or directed for distribution by your will, must go through the state's probate process before they are distributed to your heirs. Any assets for which you previously named a beneficiary, such as a life insurance policy, or an IRA, pass directly to that beneficiary without going through probate. Furthermore, the distribution of an asset with a specifically named beneficiary takes precedence over any conflicting distribution of that same asset in a will. For example, a beneficiary named on an IRA takes precedence over a designated heir for that IRA named in the will. Often, a will also names guardians and trustees for minor children. A will becomes a public document.

Revocable Living Trust

Because of the limitations of a will, some people choose to set up a revocable living trust (RLT), which can be changed over time. An RLT has the following benefits over a will:

- It can avoid court interference at incapacity and death.
- It avoids probate.
- It can consolidate assets into one trust.
- It provides maximum privacy.
- It can be changed by the grantor at any time.
- The trust can continue after your death and is managed by the trustee(s) you select.
- You control when the beneficiaries receive the assets in the trust.
- The trust can protect the assets from a beneficiary's creditors and spouse, as well as any irresponsible spending.

While a trust adds an additional expense to an estate plan, its benefits might be worth the added cost.

Incapacity Plan

An incapacity plan allows you to authorize someone you know and trust, such as a spouse, family member, or close friend, to make important healthcare and financial decisions for you in the event you become incapacitated. An incapacity plan is typically executed through the following three documents:

- **Durable Power of Attorney:** You appoint an individual who has the authority to make financial and legal decisions on your behalf according to the instructions.
- **Durable Power of Attorney for Healthcare:** You appoint an individual to communicate with your doctors, and make medical decisions on your behalf, in the event you become unable to make these decisions on your own.
- **Living Will/Health-Care Proxy:** This document communicates your final wishes for end-of-life decisions, such as life support, resuscitation, etc. (AARP provides free forms. Go to https://www.aarp.org and search "advance directive forms".)

On a side note, I have found it extremely helpful to create a personal health-care folder for my wife and me, and I highly recommend you do the same. Such a folder should include your estate planning documents (including health directives), a copy of your insurance cards, a list of doctors and pharmacies, and a list of your drugs and supplements. You should also complete a proxy-access request and authorization form, allowing your preferred caregiver access to your online electronic patient portal.[1] This authorization form may be obtained:

1. At your doctor's office
2. At a hospital
3. On a hospital's website

When formulating your estate plan, you will want to cover the following:

- [ ] Provide for your spouse/partner and minor and disabled children.
- [ ] Provide for family members with special needs without affecting earned government benefits.
- [ ] Provide for family members who are irresponsible with money, or who might need future protection from creditors or divorce.
- [ ] If the estate includes a business, create a plan to sell or transfer ownership of the business. A buy-sell agreement between/among co-owners is often used for this purpose.
- [ ] Obtain life insurance to provide survivorship income, pay off your debts, provide liquidity, equalize an estate among family members, and pay estate taxes.
- [ ] If employed, obtain disability insurance to replace income in the event of a disability.
- [ ] Obtain long-term care insurance (as discussed in Chapter 2).
- [ ] Leave instructions regarding the location of important estate planning documents, including wills, trusts, life insurance, disability insurance, long-term care policies, deeds, titles, marriage certificate, birth or adoption certificates of children, military discharge papers, and any other important documents. These instructions should also include the location of your passwords, and a list of your digital accounts, including PayPal and cryptocurrency accounts, websites, domain names, digital storage accounts, (including photos, videos, music, movies, e-books), prepaid accounts, frequent flier and other rewards accounts, social media and email accounts. (FYI, Facebook has a legacy change/memorialization setting option, which allows you to choose a legacy contact, or request that your account be permanently deleted after you die).
- [ ] Create a balance sheet listing all assets and liabilities. (See list in Chapter 3.)
- [ ] If you are still employed, have available for your loved ones an easily accessible list of all your employee benefits, including:
    - Group health insurance, dental insurance, and vision insurance
    - Group disability insurance

- Group life insurance
- Accidental death and dismemberment insurance
- Group long-term care insurance
- Qualified retirement plans, including 401(k), 403(b), profit sharing, 457 plans, SIMPLE IRA plans, SEP-IRA, and deferred compensation plans
- Non-qualified retirement plans
- Stock options and employee stock ownership plans (ESOP)
- Pension plans

All of these important documents should be stored in a safe, fire-safe box, or safe-deposit box at a location where your spouse/partner or other loved ones can easily find it.

By planning your estate now, you will be able to organize your records, locate and review titles and beneficiary designations, and find and correct errors. This will make life a lot easier, and save a lot of time and unnecessary headaches, for your spouse/partner and other heirs. Keep your plan current - a major life change, such as marriage, divorce, or the death of a spouse/partner, may necessitate changes to your estate plan, including changes to your beneficiary designations. Review your estate plan and your beneficiary designations from time to time to make sure they are all up to date. Work with a financial advisor and an estate attorney to review your estate plan. If you are not currently working with any professionals, ask your family, friends, or CPA, for a trusted referral.

What if You Become Incapacitated and Don't Have an Estate Plan?

If you become incapacitated and don't have an estate plan, your family will have no ability to control your assets, and you risk having that control in the hands of a stranger. If you are incapacitated without a plan in place, a court will appoint a conservatorship or guardianship that will control how your assets are used on your behalf. This public process can be expensive and time-consuming.[2] In addition, your family will have to make important medical decisions without knowing your wishes.

What if You Die Without an Estate Plan?

If you were to die without a valid will, your estate would be subject to the intestacy laws of the state where you live and would be distributed by a probate court. The court would distribute your property according to the state's rules of inheritance. In many states, if you are married and have children, your assets are apportioned among your spouse and children, possibly leaving your spouse with insufficient assets to live on. If you have minor children, the court could appoint a trustee to manage their inheritance. If both parents die intestate (without valid wills), the court will appoint a guardian and trustee to manage the minor children's inheritance and make decisions on their behalf; this might not be the person whom you would have chosen to care for your children.

The best time to plan your estate is NOW. In my experience, people put off estate planning for a variety of reasons. They may not want to face their own mortality or incapacity, they feel that they are too young, they feel that they don't have enough assets, they are too busy, or they just can't agree on a guardian or trustee. But it is much better to have a plan in place now, and change it later if necessary, than to have no plan at all.

CHAPTER 5:
TAXES IN RETIREMENT

Many people mistakenly assume that when they retire, their taxes will automatically decline. After all, when you stop working, your income may drop, and you stop paying Social Security and Medicare taxes. But for some retirees, their income remains the same in retirement, or even increases, because they have many sources of retirement income. They may even face additional taxes, in the form of Social Security tax, and higher Medicare premiums.

Taxation of Retirement Assets

We can divide retirement assets into four tax buckets:

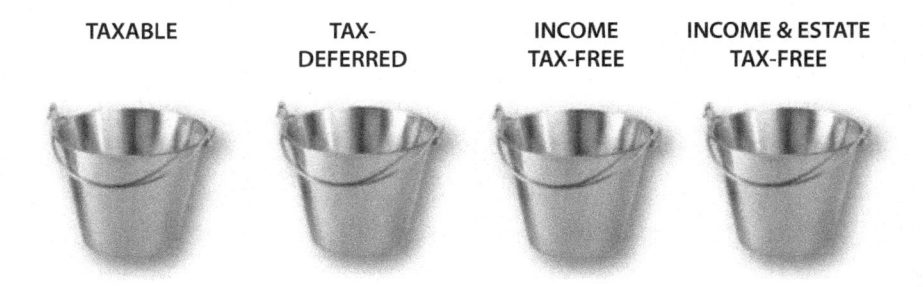

TAXABLE	TAX-DEFERRED	INCOME TAX-FREE	INCOME & ESTATE TAX-FREE

1. **The Taxable Bucket:** This represents accounts that produce 1099 forms, such as bank accounts and brokerage accounts. These taxable accounts might hold CDs, money markets, savings/checking accounts, stocks, bonds, commodities, mutual funds, exchange traded funds (ETFs), real estate investment trusts (REITs), real estate, and other income-producing assets.

2. **The Tax-Deferred Bucket:** This represents qualified retirement accounts such as 401(k), 403(b), 457(b), Profit-Sharing, SIMPLE IRA, and Simplified Employee Pensions (SEP), as well as Traditional IRAs. This also includes non-qualified retirement accounts, such as Deferred Compensation Plans, Executive Bonus Plans, Group Carve-Out

Plans, and Split-Dollar Life Insurance. This bucket also includes savings bonds and annuities, which can be "qualified" annuities (funded with pre-tax contributions) or "non-qualified" annuities (funded with after-tax contributions). Note: these accounts can be funded with the same type of assets referenced in the taxable bucket, but are now tax-deferred (not subject to taxation until withdrawals are taken), because they are held in these tax-advantaged accounts.

3. **Income Tax-Free Bucket:** Roth IRAs are income tax-free if certain conditions are met (discussed below). Contributions to a Roth IRA are made with after-tax dollars and can be withdrawn at any time without taxes or penalties. Withdrawals of Roth IRA earnings are also tax and penalty-free, but only if you have had the account for at least 5 years and the withdrawals are not taken until age 59½ or later. You can also avoid tax penalties under other conditions; visit https://www.irs.gov/taxtopics/tc557 or speak to your tax professional. Note: these accounts can be funded with the same type of assets referenced in the taxable bucket, but are now tax-deferred and possibly tax-free, if certain conditions are met, because they are held in these tax-advantaged accounts. Municipal bond interest can also provide tax-free income in retirement and should be held in a taxable account (not in a tax-deferred account or a Roth IRA, which negate the tax benefits). A life insurance death benefit is also normally paid out income tax-free.

4. **Income and Estate Tax-Free Bucket:** This includes life insurance that is properly owned, such that the proceeds are not includable in the insured's estate. For example, the policy might be owned by adult children or by an Irrevocable Life Insurance Trust (ILIT). Life insurance in combination with an ILIT is often used for estate planning purposes for larger estates; charitable trusts are often used as well.

Prior to retirement, most people hold a majority of their assets in the tax-deferred bucket. This has the potential to create significant tax liabilities in retirement, when people typically start to make withdrawals from that "bucket," and the "deferred" taxes become due. To reduce future heavy tax liability, it sometimes makes more financial sense to spend down those assets prior to retirement, or to re-allocate those assets over time into the tax-free bucket. An example of this is a Roth conversion, in which you transfer assets from a tax-deferred account, such as a traditional IRA or 401(k), to a

Roth IRA. (Please keep in mind that ordinary federal and state income taxes are due in the year of the conversion.) This option may be worth considering for those in a lower income tax bracket, or if you think that tax rates will increase in the future. Roth IRA conversions will be discussed further in this chapter.

Sources of Retirement Income

Next, let's discuss sources of retirement income. These include:

- Social Security benefits
- Pensions
- Earned income
- Qualified retirement plan distributions
- Traditional IRA distributions
- Roth IRA distributions
- Annuity distributions
- Real estate rental income
- Withdrawals from taxable accounts

Many of these income sources are taxed annually as ordinary income, including:

- Social Security (whether this is taxable depends on your total household income)
- Pensions
- Earned income
- Qualified retirement plan distributions
- Traditional IRA distributions
- Annuity distributions
- Real estate rental income

Withdrawals from taxable accounts, such as a savings or brokerage account, are not taxable. What triggers a tax on these accounts is the *earnings*, such as the interest earned in a savings account and the dividends and capital gains earned in a brokerage account. These dividends and capital gains are taxable, whether reinvested or paid in cash. Furthermore, these earnings are taxed in different ways:

- Earned interest from savings accounts, money markets, CDs, and many bonds are taxed as ordinary income in the year they are earned.
- Qualified dividends and long-term capital gains are taxed at capital gains rates.
- Non-qualified dividends and short-term capital gains are taxed as ordinary income.
- Interest earned on municipal bonds is exempt from federal income taxes and may also be exempt from state and local taxes.
- Interest earned on treasury securities, such as treasury bills and bonds, is exempt from state and local taxes, but is fully taxable at the federal level.
- Capital gains from the sale of municipal or treasury securities are taxable.

Roth IRA distributions are tax and penalty-free under each of the following circumstances:

- Withdrawals of contributions are always tax free because the account is funded with after-tax money.
- The withdrawal of earnings is tax and penalty free if the participant is at least 59½ years old, and the IRA has been open for at least 5 years.
- The distributions of inherited Roth IRAs are tax and penalty free.

If you have multiple sources of retirement income to choose from, you have several important decisions to make, including:

- Which income source should you draw from first?

- When should you start taking Social Security income?
- When should you start taking distributions from your IRAs and qualified retirement plans?

Every individual's circumstances are different, so factors such as age, health, total income and investments, tax bracket, and income needs will determine the answers to these questions.

Federal Income Tax

Below are the 2020 federal income tax brackets. Some people mistakenly think that, if their total taxable income falls within the range listed under a particular bracket, all that income is taxed at that one rate. But in the U.S., income is taxed on a progressive scale, such that only the portion of taxable income that falls within a particular bracket is taxed at that bracket's rate. For example, for a married couple filing jointly with a household taxable income of $80,000, the first $19,400 of taxable income is taxed at 10%, the next $59,549 ($78,950 - $19,401) is taxed at 12%, and the final $1,049 ($80,000 - $78,951) is taxed at 22%. So, although the marginal tax bracket is 22% (because the total income is $80,000), the actual or effective tax rate is much less than 22%; in fact, it is closer to 12%. (Tax brackets are based on taxable income, which is gross income minus eligible deductions.)

Federal Tax Brackets for 2020

Tax Rate	Single	Married Filing Jointly	Married Filing Separately	Head of Household
10%	$0-$9,700	$0-$19,400	$0-$9,700	$0-$13,850
12%	$9,701-$39,475	$19,401-$78,950	$9,701-$39,475	$13,851-$52,850
22%	$39,476-$84,200	$78,951-$168,400	$39,476-$84,200	$52,851-$84,200
24%	$84,201-$160,725	$168,401-$321,450	$84,201-$160,725	$84,201-$160,700
32%	$160,726-$204,100	$321,451-$408,200	$160,726-$204,100	$160,701-$204,100
35%	$204,101-$510,300	$408,201-$612,350	$204,101-$306,175	$204,101-$510,300
37%	Over $510,300	Over $612,350	Over $306,175	Over $510,300

Standard Deduction or Itemized Deductions?

When filing your tax return, you may claim the standard deduction or itemize your deductions to lower your taxable income and your tax liability. The standard deduction lowers your taxable income by a fixed amount (see table below), while itemized deductions are eligible expenses that can be claimed. You can choose whichever method lowers your tax bill the most.

The 2020 Standard Deduction

Filing Status	Standard Deduction
Single	$12,400
Married Filing Jointly	$24,800
Married Filing Separately	$12,400
Head of Household	$18,650

The standard deduction is increased by $1,300 for those age 65 or older, and for those who are blind. If you are unmarried and not a surviving spouse, the deduction is increased by $1,650. If someone can claim you as a dependent, you get a smaller standard deduction.

Most people benefit most by taking the standard deduction, especially since state taxes and local property taxes have been capped at $10,000.

Capital Gains

Next, let's discuss the tax ramifications of capital gains. Capital gains are triggered when investment assets and real property are sold at a profit. Capital gains on investments and real estate that are held for one year or less are taxed as ordinary income. Capital gains on investments and real estate that are held for a year and a day or longer are taxed as long-term capital gains. Like ordinary income, capital gains are taxed on a progressive scale. Depending on your taxable income and marital status, long-term capital gains are taxed at the rate of 0%, 15% or 20% (see table on next page). Qualified dividends are taxed under long-term capital gains rates, while non-qualified dividends are taxed as ordinary income.

Dividend and Long-Term Capital Gains Brackets for 2020

Long-Term Capital Gains Tax Rate	Single	Married Filing Jointly	Married Filing Separately	Head of Household
0%	$0-$40,000	$0-$80,000	$0-$40,000	$0-$53,600
15%	$40,001-$441,450	$80,001-$496,600	$40,001-$248,300	$53,601-$469,050
20%	Over $441,450	Over $496,600	Over $248,300	Over $469,050

Some people believe that capital gains are realized only upon the sale of a capital asset that has appreciated in value. But you can be liable for capital gains from a mutual fund you own, even if you never sell it. This is because of "phantom" gains. For example, let's say that Mutual Fund X bought Apple stock in 2010. You invest in Mutual Fund X at the end of 2018 and continue to hold it. In the beginning of 2019, the fund manager of Mutual Fund X decides to sell all of its Apple stock shares at a significant gain. Any gain recognized on the sale of a stock must be passed through to the current shareholders, regardless of how long they have owned the shares. So be aware that, if you hold mutual funds in a taxable account, you will likely recognize capital gains in most years, even during years in which your mutual funds drop in value; you cannot control phantom gains. Therefore, it pays to be informed and to understand which type of account is best to hold a particular investment. You might be better off holding mutual funds and bonds in tax-deferred accounts, and holding more tax-efficient assets, such as exchange traded funds (ETFs) and individual stocks, in taxable accounts.

3.8% Net Investment Income Tax

In addition to income tax and capital gains tax, some people must also pay the Net Investment Income Tax (NIIT) on certain income. For individuals with an adjusted gross income (AGI) of over $200,000, married filing jointly with an AGI of over $250,000, married filing separately with an AGI of over $125,000, and head of household with an AGI of over $200,000, the 3.8% NIIT is imposed on the following income:

- Interest
- Dividends

- Capital gains
- Rental and royalty income
- Non-qualified annuity payments
- Certain business income, including passive income

Under some circumstances, certain estates and trusts are also subject to this income tax. For more information, please visit https://www.irs.gov/newsroom/questions-and-answers-on-the-net-investment-income-tax, or speak to your tax professional.

Required Minimum Distributions

Next, let's discuss Required Minimum Distributions (RMDs). Some people have a large portion of their retirement money in qualified retirement accounts and traditional IRAs. Generally, most, if not all, of their contributions are made with pre-tax dollars, which means that most, if not all, of their distributions will be subject to ordinary income tax. Under the current tax laws, you must begin taking RMDs when you turn age 72. (If you reached age 70½ prior to January 1, 2020, then your RMD age is 70½ years old). There is an exception to this rule. If you are still working, and you're not an owner of more than 5% of the company you work for, some qualified retirement plans, such as 401(k) plans, 403(b) plans, and 457(b) plans, may allow you to defer taking RMDs until you are no longer working. Check with your employer to see if their plan allows you to defer RMDs. Also, speak to your tax professional to determine if you qualify for this exception. Only current employment is relevant here; qualified retirement plans from prior employment (and IRAs) don't qualify for the RMD exception.

What is the Latest Date to Take Your First RMD?

Once required to be taken, RMDs must be taken annually. Except for your first RMD, you must take the RMD by the end of each calendar year. For your initial RMD, you have until April 1st of the year following the year you turn age 72. For example, if you celebrated your 72nd birthday on January 1, 2020, you would have until April 1, 2021 to take your first RMD. But, just because you can delay taking your initial RMD until the following year, should you? That depends on your income and tax status. If you delay taking your initial RMD until the following year, you will be taking two RMDs in one year - because you still have to take the annual RMD for the following year, and that could impact your taxes for that following year. One reason to delay the initial RMD until the following year is if you expect your income to drop in the following year. For example, if you are planning to retire at or near the end of the year you turn 72, but you work for most of that year, it might pay to delay the RMD to the following year, when you have less taxable income. You should make this calculation to determine your tax liability under both scenarios – taking the initial RMD in the current year versus delaying it to the next year and having to take two RMDs that year.

What is the Formula for Calculating Your RMD?

The formula for calculating the amount of your RMD for each of your qualified investment accounts is: the account balance at the end of the prior year, divided by your remaining life expectancy (as listed in the Uniform Lifetime Table). For example, assume that the year-end account balance on your traditional IRA for the year prior to you turning 72 was $500,000. Under the Uniform Lifetime table (below), the remaining life expectancy for age 72 is 25.6 years. $500,000 divided by 25.6 = $19,531.25. So, for this example, your first RMD would be $19,531.25. To calculate the RMDs at other ages, use the figures from the table below.

RMD Uniform Lifetime Table

Age	Distribution Period	Age	Distribution Period	Age	Distribution Period	Age	Distribution Period	Age	Distribution Period
70	27.4	80	18.7	90	11.4	100	6.3	110	3.1
71	26.5	81	17.9	91	10.8	101	5.9	111	2.9
72	25.6	82	17.1	92	10.2	102	5.5	112	2.6
73	24.7	83	16.3	93	9.6	103	5.2	113	2.4
74	23.8	84	15.5	94	9.1	104	4.9	114	2.1
75	22.9	85	14.8	95	8.6	105	4.5	115+	1.9
76	22.0	86	14.1	96	8.1	106	4.2		
77	21.2	87	13.4	97	7.6	107	3.9		
78	20.3	88	12.7	98	7.1	108	3.7		
79	19.5	89	12.0	99	6.7	109	3.4		

Under certain circumstances, a different life expectancy table is used to calculate your RMD. If your spouse is the sole beneficiary on the account, and is more than 10 years younger than you, you would calculate your RMD using the joint life and last survivor expectancy table, known as Life Expectancy Table II or Joint Life Expectancy Table. (Please see https://www.fidelity.com/bin-public/060_www_fidelity_com/documents/Joint-Life-Expectancy-Table.pdf). In this situation, you would not be required to withdraw as much money as you would if your spouse were older. Though the RMD calculation method remains the same, you must first obtain the dividing variable from the Life Expectancy II Table using your age and your spouse's age. Another resource is the IRS IRA Required Minimum Distribution Worksheet at: https://www.irs.gov/pub/irs-tege/jlls_rmd_worksheet.pdf. You might also want to speak to your tax professional.

Obviously, as age increases, life expectancy decreases. That does not mean, however, that the amount of your annual RMDs decreases. On the contrary, as you age, the percentage you must withdraw from your retirement account(s) increases. For example, assuming the year-end value of your traditional IRA is $500,000 at age 70 and at age 75. At age 70, your RMD would be $18,248.18 ($500,000 balance divided by 27.4 life expectancy), or 3.65%. At age 75, your RMD would be $21,834.06 ($500,000 divided by 22.9), or 4.37%. You can calculate the percentage of your distribution for any given year by dividing 100 by the life expectancy factor for that year. In the example above, you divide 100 by 27.4 (the life expectancy for age 70), which equals 3.65%; 100 divided by 22.9 (the life expectancy for age 75) is 4.37%.

For ease of reference, some other age distribution rates are:

- Age 80: 5.34%
- Age 85: 6.76%
- Age 90: 8.77%

(These ever-increasing distribution rates can become a big problem if you suffer stock market losses early in retirement, creating a sequence of return risk, which will be discussed later in Chapter 9).

Other than the first year you qualify (when you have the option to delay), it is extremely important that you take the RMD each year. The failure to take your annual RMD results in a 50% tax penalty. Using the earlier example where your initial RMD at age 72 is $19,531.25, the failure to take it would result in a tax penalty of $9,765.63, and you would still be required to take that year's RMD. The IRS could waive all or part of the penalty for reasonable errors, which include bad or incorrect advice from a financial advisor, an illness, a death in the family, or an address change that disrupts communication from the firm holding your IRA or qualified retirement plan.[1] The institution that holds your investment accounts, and/or your financial advisor, should remind you to take your RMD, but you should still pay attention to the deadlines.

What if you have different types of retirement plans, such as a 401(k) and an IRA, can you combine the amounts from those different accounts, and take just one RMD? The answer is no; you must take a separate RMD from each of those plans. Even though a 401(k) and an IRA are both retirement plans, they are not the same type of account, and are treated differently, so they cannot be combined. What if you have two IRAs; can you take the combined RMDs from one account? This time, the answer is yes because they are the same type of account. If you are married, each spouse must take RMDs from their respective IRAs or qualified retirement accounts. Please note, that if you more than satisfy your RMD one year by taking a distribution that is higher than your required minimum amount, you cannot use the excess distribution as a credit towards the next year. Every year stands on its own, and you must calculate and take the appropriate RMD.

Social Security Taxation

If your only source of income is Social Security, you are not subject to federal income tax. If you have other sources of income, your Social Security income might be taxable up to 85% (higher income households), or possibly not at all (lower income households). The formula to determine how much of your Social Security income is taxable is based on something called "provisional income".

Provisional Income

Provisional income equals 50% of your Social Security income plus ordinary income plus dividends and capital gains plus non-taxable interest from municipal bonds (Roth IRA distributions are not included in provisional income).

Social Security Tax Thresholds

Single:	Married Filing Jointly:
$25,000 (50%)	$32,000 (50%)
$34,000 (85%)	$44,000 (85%)

If you are single, and your provisional income is less than $25,000, none of your Social Security income is subject to federal income tax. If your provisional income falls between $25,000 and just under $34,000, up to 50% of your Social Security income is subject to federal income tax. If your provisional income is $34,000 or higher, up to 85% of your Social Security income is subject to federal income tax.

If you are married filing jointly, and your provisional income is less than $32,000, none of your Social Security income is subject to federal income tax. If your provisional income falls between $32,000 and just under $44,000, up to 50% of your Social Security income is subject to federal income tax. If your provisional income is $44,000 or higher, up to 85% of your Social Security income is subject to federal income tax.

I have included two examples of how to calculate tax on Social Security income. In both scenarios, the households are married, filing jointly and have a total income of $60,000.

Example 1: $20,000 Social Security Income + $40,000 IRA withdrawal = $60,000 total income

- **Step 1, Provisional Income Calculation:** $20,000 Social Security income x 50% = $10,000, + ordinary income $40,000, + dividends and capital gains $0, + non-taxable interest from municipal bonds $0, = provisional income of $50,000.

- **Step 2, First Threshold Calculation:** Provisional income $50,000 - first threshold $32,000 = $18,000. Next, multiply $18,000 x 50% = $9,000.

- **Step 3, Second Threshold Calculation:** Provisional income $50,000 - second threshold ($44,000) = $6,000. Next, multiply $6,000 x 35% (85% - 50% that has already been calculated) = $2,100.

- **Step 4, Taxable Social Security Benefit:** First threshold $9,000 + second threshold $2,100 = taxable Social Security of $11,100, which is 55% of the total Social Security benefit.

Flowchart for Example 1: $20,000 Social Security with $40,000 IRA withdrawal = $60,000 total income

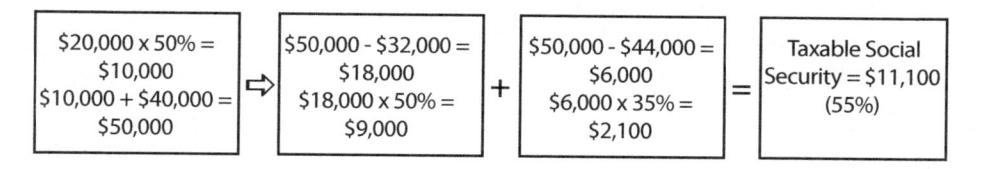

| $20,000 x 50% = $10,000 $10,000 + $40,000 = $50,000 | ⇨ | $50,000 - $32,000 = $18,000 $18,000 x 50% = $9,000 | + | $50,000 - $44,000 = $6,000 $6,000 x 35% = $2,100 | = | Taxable Social Security = $11,100 (55%) |

Example 2: $40,000 Social Security income + $20,000 IRA withdrawal = $60,000 total income.

- **Step 1, Provisional Income Calculation:** $40,000 Social Security income x 50% = $20,000, + ordinary income $20,000, + dividends and capital gains $0, + non-taxable interest from municipal bonds $0, = provisional income of $40,000.

- **Step 2, First Threshold Calculation:** Provisional income $40,000 - first threshold $32,000 = $8,000. Next, multiply $8,000 x 50% = $4,000.

- **Step 3, Second Threshold Calculation:** Provisional income $40,000 - second threshold $44,000 = -$4,000. Since the second threshold is negative, there is no additional tax threshold.

- **Step 4, Taxable Social Security Benefit:** First threshold $4,000 + second threshold $0 = taxable Social Security of $4,000, which is 10% of the Social Security benefit.

Flowchart for Example 2: $40,000 Social Security with $20,000 IRA withdrawal = $60,000 total income

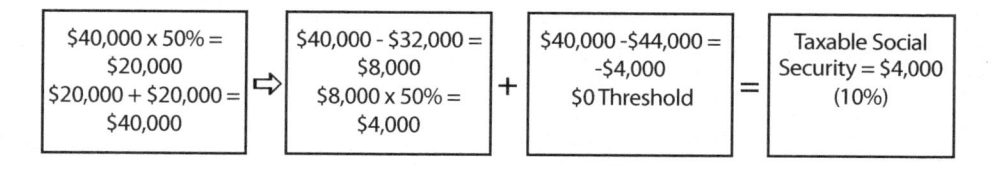

| $40,000 x 50% = $20,000 $20,000 + $20,000 = $40,000 | ⇨ | $40,000 - $32,000 = $8,000 $8,000 x 50% = $4,000 | + | $40,000 - $44,000 = -$4,000 $0 Threshold | = | Taxable Social Security = $4,000 (10%) |

As you can see, even though the Social Security income is higher in the second example, a smaller portion of the Social Security income is taxable because of the provisional income determination. Remember, other sources of income are what cause your Social Security benefits to become taxable.

Taxation of Annuities

Annuities are often purchased to supplement other sources of retirement income. Annuities can either be "qualified" (funded with pre-tax dollars) or "non-qualified" (funded with after-tax dollars). During the deferral period (before distributions are taken), both qualified and non-qualified annuities grow tax-deferred, meaning that no taxes on earnings are reported or due. During the distribution period (when distributions are taken), qualified and non-qualified annuities are taxed differently. With a qualified annuity, just like an IRA or any retirement plan funded with pre-tax dollars, all distributions are taxed as ordinary income. With non-qualified annuities, the earnings portion of the distributions is taxable as ordinary income. When distributions are taken, earnings are considered on the last in, first out method. In other words, the earnings portion comes out first, and then your cost basis (the amount that you paid into the annuity), comes out next. This is not very tax efficient since all earnings come out first. However, if you annuitize your non-qualified annuity, whereby you exchange with the insurance company the rights to the annuity's cash value in return for regular payments for a specified period or for life, then those payments will be based on an "exclusion ratio". Because annuitization payments include both earnings and your cost basis, the full amount of the payments are not taxable. Once your cost basis is exhausted, then all future payments are considered earnings, and taxed as ordinary income. If a withdrawal is taken from a non-qualified annuity before age 59½, there could be a 10% penalty tax on the earnings portion. For a qualified annuity, the full withdrawal might be subject to a 10% penalty if taken before age 59½. (As with distributions from IRAs and qualified retirement accounts, there are exceptions to these rules but that is beyond the scope of this book - please speak to your tax professional.)

Strategies for Tax Control

Now that we have discussed taxes in retirement, you may be wondering how you can improve your tax situation. Here are some factors to consider:

- Be aware of how different sources of income can affect your overall income tax. This includes Social Security, pension income, annuity income, distributions from IRAs and qualified retirement plans, and capital gains and dividends. A tax professional or financial advisor should be able to help you calculate your future tax liability using tax-planning software.

- Understand which type of account is best to hold a particular investment. For example, you may be better off holding mutual funds and bonds in tax-deferred accounts, and holding more tax-efficient assets, such as exchange traded funds (ETFs) and individual stocks, in taxable accounts.

- Consider selling investments with losses to offset capital gains in your non-retirement accounts. For the sale of an investment to be considered a loss and not a "wash sale", you cannot buy back the same investment within 30 days, but you can buy an investment with similar exposure, through an ETF, for example. This strategy is known as tax-loss harvesting. You can use up to $3,000 of capital losses to offset earned income.

- Don't waste your deductions. As previously discussed, under the current tax laws, most people are more likely to take the standard deduction, instead of itemizing their expenses. Again, the standard deduction is $12,400 for single filers and $24,800 for married filers. The standard deduction is $1,300 higher for those who are over 65 or blind; and $1,650 higher if also unmarried and not a surviving spouse. So, for example, a married couple, both age 65 or older and filing jointly, would have a total standard deduction of $27,400 ($24,800 + $2,600). If this couple's only source of income is Social Security in the amount of $40,000, they would pay no federal income taxes. Now assume they own traditional IRAs, and take distributions totaling $22,269, increasing their total income to $62,269. Because of their standard deduction (and the combination of Social Security income and IRA distributions), they would not incur any federal income taxes, up to this income. The point is that if you can take IRA distributions and incur little to no federal income taxes, you should take advantage of the standard deduction. Since you can't carry your deductions forward, if you don't use them to your advantage, they are wasted forever!

- Don't wait until age 72 to take distributions from your IRAs or qualified retirement plans. Conventional thinking says that, if you don't need the income before then, you should delay taking distributions on your IRAs and qualified retirement plans until you reach age 72. But, just because you can defer your distributions until then, should you? Not necessarily, it depends on your total income and your sources of income. In the previous example, it makes sense to take the distributions earlier because doing so will not trigger federal income taxes. Deferring distributions from your IRAs and qualified retirement plans may cause you to pay higher taxes on your Social Security income later and may also increase your Medicare premiums, if the distributions result in higher income. In addition, if your tax-deferred bucket of money continues to grow, your future RMDs will be higher, which could cause you to pay higher taxes later. So, if your overall income is lower in retirement, it may be better to start taking distributions earlier than age 72, even if you don't need the income.

If you don't need the income from your traditional IRA, consider doing one or more of the following:

1. Do a Roth conversion. If you don't need the income from your traditional IRA, instead of taking the distribution, you can convert your traditional IRA to a Roth IRA. Even if the Roth conversion causes you to owe a small amount in taxes, this may still be advantageous to do. The benefits of the Roth IRA are:

    - Withdrawals are tax and penalty free if you wait 5 years to take a distribution and you are at least age 59½ years old.
    - Withdrawals don't count towards your provisional income for Social Security taxation.
    - Roth IRAs are not subject to RMDs.

2. Use the IRA distributions to buy long-term care insurance.

3. Use the IRA distributions to buy permanent life insurance. The benefits of permanent life insurance are:

    - The death benefit provides instant liquidity.
    - The death benefit is normally income tax-free, making it a tax-efficient asset to pass to heirs. For a large estate, it may be necessary to have the life insurance owned by an Irrevocable Life Insurance Trust (ILIT) or by adult children to avoid estate taxation.

These strategies should be discussed with your tax advisor or other financial professional. This information is general in nature and should not be considered tax advice.

Although identifying tax opportunities is important, this undertaking should be done within the context of an overall financial plan. If you are likely to spend most of your assets during your lifetime, tax-efficiency should be viewed as secondary to meeting your retirement goals. On the other hand, if you expect to have a large amount of funds left over at the end of your lifetime, leaving tax-efficient assets, such as a Roth IRA or life insurance, would likely be more advantageous to your beneficiaries than leaving a traditional IRA or qualified retirement plan.

CHAPTER 6:
BAD ADVICE, SCAMS, FRAUD, AND IDENTITY THEFT

This chapter deals with the financial risks of receiving bad advice, scams, fraud, and identity theft, and provides some suggestions on how to find good advice.

Bad Advice, Scams, and Fraud

Bad advice can come from a financial professional, a family member, a friend, or anyone else that gives you financial advice. Often, family members and friends will hear of a "hot tip" about a "sure thing that can't miss," and are eager to tell everyone about it. These tips don't often pan out. While most financial professionals are honest, provide good advice, and put their client's interests ahead of their own, as in any profession, there are always some bad seeds who are only looking out for their own interests. There are countless stories about financial "professionals" churning their client's accounts (needlessly buying and selling assets to generate commissions and fees), selling their clients unsuitable investments or insurance products, using clients' assets for personal use, or running a Ponzi scheme (Bernie Madoff being the worst of the worst). These con artists are often "fast talkers," and many are very polished. They often promise high returns with little or no risk. They may even believe their own BS. They often have deft skill sets in the paper chase and litigation stalling game and take advantage of the legal system. The federal statute of limitations on financial crimes is five years. Unfortunately, many people don't realize they have been defrauded until several years have passed, and often after the statute of limitations has run out. Legal proceedings often take several years. By the time that prosecutors decide on proceeding with the case, time is almost up, and they will often cease their case knowing that they are up against the statue.[1]

The Modern Con Artist Often...[2]

- Establish themselves with "solid" investments and a history of payments
- Partners with credible professionals in the financial industry
- Insulate themselves from lawsuits by working with many notable attorneys in the area
- Uses official-looking documents that appear legitimate
- Produces multiple entities among which they can move money
- Changes business locations and business names
- Offers seemingly viable explanations to clients to bide more time with their money
- Uses the legal system to their advantage.

Be aware of the following red flags:

- Promises of high returns with little or no risk
- Overly consistent returns
- Unregistered investment products
- Unlicensed and unregistered sellers

Good Advice

As stated earlier, I do believe that most financial professionals are honest, and provide good advice. So how do you recognize good advice from bad?

- Don't take any financial advice you receive as gospel (especially if it's an absolute statement).
- Work with an advisor who is a fiduciary, a professional who is required to put your interests above their own. If you don't know if your advisor is a fiduciary, just ask.
- Make sure the advice you are getting is specific to your individual situation, and not a "cookie cutter" approach.
- If something sounds too good to be true, it probably is.

- Diversify your investments. Don't put all your eggs in one basket, no matter how good an investment sounds.

- Make sure you understand what you are investing in or buying. Annuities and insurance products can be complex and contain many "moving parts". If the advisor struggles to explain a product to you, chances are, they don't understand it.

- Before meeting with a prospective financial advisor, check his/her background on https://brokercheck.finra.org/. This report tells you whether the advisor has been involved in any customer complaints or arbitrations, regulatory actions, employment terminations, bankruptcy filings, and criminal or civil judicial proceedings. It also notes your advisor's professional licenses, the states of licensure, and past employers.

Prior to hiring a financial advisor, you may want to ask the following questions:

- What services do you offer? Do you offer financial planning? Do you offer investment management? Do you sell insurance and annuity products?

- What is your process when working with new clients?

- How will you manage my money?

- Where will my money be held?

- How do you measure success?

- How do you get paid? (Advisors are typically compensated for their time on an hourly or flat fee basis, or they receive a percentage of the assets under management, a commission on products sold, or a combination of these methods.)

- What is your background, experience, and credentials?

- How often will we speak or meet? How quickly will you get back to me if I call or send an email?

- What is your succession plan?

A financial advisor should act like a coach and a teacher, by providing education and giving you advice. A financial advisor should not act like a salesperson and should not push financial products on you. During the initial meeting, the advisor should ask you many questions to determine if and how they can help you, and what your financial goals are. They should be gathering the necessary information that will enable them to develop a plan and specific recommendations for you. If the advisor begins peddling investment or insurance products in your first meeting, leave the meeting and don't return, as this advisor is more interested in selling you a product and making a commission, and less interested in your financial well-being.

Identity Theft

Some people believe that their home, their business, their investments, or their personal assets are their most valuable and sought-after asset. But in reality, your most important asset is your personal data. "This data is a highly sought-after commodity that is widely traded. Every day, people throughout the world give away large amounts of very personal and valuable information about themselves. How? They do a Google search, buy something from Amazon, surf Facebook, or just turn their iPhones on."[3] Many people do not realize how much their lives are invaded each day. Identity theft can be devastating to an individual, and it's becoming more common. "Nearly 60 Million Americans have been affected by identity theft, according to a 2018 online survey by the Harris Poll."[4] Identity theft takes many forms: someone steals your credit card information, and uses it to make purchases; someone steals your Social Security number, driver's license number and/or other personally identifiable information (PII) to fraudulently apply for credit, open new accounts, get a tax refund, or use medical services, to name a few. This can damage your credit status and cost you time and money to clear your name and restore your credit.

If you suspect that your identity has been stolen, here are 10 steps that you can take to minimize the damage:[5]

- File a report with the Federal Trade Commission.
- Contact your local police department.
- Notify the IRS and your identity theft insurance, if applicable.
- Place a fraud alert on your credit reports.
- Freeze your credit.
- Sign up for a credit monitoring service.

- Tighten security on your accounts.
- Review your credit reports for mystery accounts.
- Review credit card and bank statements for unauthorized charges.
- Close current credit card and financial accounts and open new accounts.

Guard Your Credit and Your Identity

To guard your credit and your identity, consider the following actions:

- Freeze your credit. This is a highly effective way to prevent an identity thief from taking out credit in your name, because it restricts access to your credit reports. Lenders are unlikely to approve loans if they are unable to see a credit report. A credit freeze does not affect your credit score, and, even if frozen, your credit can still be monitored. Furthermore, you can unfreeze your credit at any time, even if only for just a few days to give a creditor time to run a report; you can even request an automatic re-freeze after a specific period of time. To freeze your credit, you must request a security freeze through each of the three nationwide credit agencies, either online or by phone.

Credit Agencies

1. **Equifax:** 800-685-1111, https://www.equifax.com/personal/: Towards the lower end of the web page, click: *Place or Manage a Freeze,* then: *Get Started With A Freeze*, and then complete the registration.
2. **Experian:** 888-397-3742, https://www.experian.com/: Under Support, click: *Security Freeze,* then *Add a security freeze,* then *Freeze my own credit file,* then complete the *Add a security freeze* page and click *submit.*
3. **TransUnion:** 888-909-8872, https://www.transunion.com/: At the top of the web page, click: *Credit Help,* then *Credit Freeze,* then under *Freeze My Credit,* click *Add Freeze,* then complete the registration and submit your request.

- Sign up for a credit-monitoring service. There are many credit-monitoring services, some of which include identity theft insurance. There is normally a cost for these services. Credit Karma (https://www.creditkarma.com/) offers a free credit-monitoring service. It monitors your TransUnion and Equifax credit reports and provides credit scores at no cost. (It does not monitor your Experian credit report or provide its score.)

- Give out your date of birth and Social Security number only when absolutely necessary. It amazes me that doctors' offices ask for your Social Security number when they don't need it.

- Shred anything containing your name, including credit card applications, credit and bank statements, and receipts. A micro-cut shredder is best, followed by a cross-cut shredder; a strip-cut shredder offers the lowest security.

- Don't give any sensitive personal information over the phone, especially if you received the phone call out of the blue. The Social Security Administration and the IRS will never call you; they will send a letter. Normally, legitimate companies and organizations will not call you to obtain personal information. Be aware of telephone scammers posing as technology providers or financial institutions and asking for login information or passwords. Again, trusted companies will not ask you for this information by phone.

- Don't answer phone calls if you are unfamiliar with the caller's number. Some of these calls are coming from overseas, and you might be charged for the phony call.

- Watch out for "phishing," which is an attempt by someone disguised as a trustworthy business to obtain personal sensitive information by electronic communication, often for malicious reasons. Cybercriminals are looking to steal your passwords, identity, credit card data, money, and personal computer files. Phishing can include:

    - Ransomware: When you click on a link or open an attachment in a fraudulent electronic communication, such as an email, and it runs a script on your computer/laptop and locks all your files. Your files are then "held for ransom" - they can't be opened without a payment to the scammer.

    - Spear phishing: These are highly targeted emails that appear to come from a familiar or trusted source, such as a friend or family member, and seek personal or confidential information.

(In either case, don't click on fake links in these electronic communications. Links that at first glance appear to be legitimate are often misspelled and contain poor grammar.)

- Be careful of cell phone threats. You might also receive text messages seeking personal information. Don't click on the links provided or reply to the texts. Just delete them.

- Immediately delete emails from senders you are unfamiliar with. Don't open attachments or click on links unless you were expecting the email. You can hover your cursor over an electronic link to verify that the address is legitimate and relates to the content of the email. Even if you are familiar with the sender, if the email looks suspicious, call the sender to verify that they sent the email. Email accounts are often hacked and can appear to be legitimate. Be aware of poor spelling or grammar and vague wording in the message.

- Never give any personal or confidential information over the internet unless you are on a secure site. A secure site contains "https" in its web address – the "s" stands for "secure." The address might also contain a padlock icon up front, indicating that it is secure.

- Don't believe promises of money or prizes.

- Don't give money or personal information to unknown charities.

- Never send money when it is requested by phone or email. There are many such scams that appear to be legitimate.

- Don't email personal information to others.

- Don't store passwords on your computer.

- Don't share passwords with other people.

- Install protective security software, including anti-virus, which protects your computer from malicious attacks, and anti-spyware, which keeps people from monitoring your activity. Security software scans your computer files, offers virus protection, and protects you from malicious attacks.

- Don't use unsecure, free, public wi-fi on your laptop or cell phone when you are in a public place. Use your own hotspot or Virtual Private Network (VPN) instead. Do not turn on the wi-fi "auto-connect" feature on your laptop or cell phone.

- Use a computer privacy screen when viewing personal information on your laptop in a public area, such as a coffee shop, airplane, train, or bus. You never know who is looking at your computer screen.

- Keep your cell phone locked when not in use and set the screen timeout to a short period of time when it is in use. Choose a secure password (one that is not easily guessed; don't use a birthdate) for your phone and other devices.

- Never leave your cell phone or laptop unattended. Don't leave your mobile device in plain sight in your car. If you must leave an electronic device in your car, lock it in your trunk before you reach your destination.

- Guard your USB drives. They should also be encrypted, and password protected.

- Don't plug an unknown USB drive into your computer.

- When not in use, keep your computer's camera covered.

- Don't use public computers, copiers, or fax machines, including hotel business centers, for personal or sensitive matters.

- When you get a new credit card in the mail, immediately sign the back. Keep your card private.

- Notify companies that you do business with of any changes to your address.

- Sign up for fraud alerts with the financial institutions that you do business with.

I realize that this chapter provides a great deal of information aimed at protecting your finances. As with suggestions made in other sections in the book, you may want to start slowly, make a few changes at first, and then make additional changes in the future.

CHAPTER 7:
LONGEVITY RISK

The remainder of this book discusses various retirement income risks and investment risks faced by pre-retirees and retirees. We'll start with longevity risk.

Longevity risk is the risk of outliving one's assets, which could result in a lower standard of living or the need to return to the workforce. As noted in Chapter 1, as life expectancies continue to increase, so does the risk of outliving your money. This is especially true for those in good health, who are expected to live longer than the average population. Half of the population will outlive their median life expectancy, some by many years. No wonder there are more 50 to 65-year-old people who fear outliving their assets (70%) than fear dying (30%).[1]

As mentioned earlier, one of the first steps to developing a retirement income plan is to take a full and accurate assessment of your assets (what you own), your liabilities (what you owe), your living expenses, and your potential sources of retirement income. Next, you'll want to "crunch" the numbers to determine if you will have enough assets and income to meet your retirement goals.

After taking an accurate assessment of your assets and liabilities, review your living expenses, and break them down into "essential" living expenses - rent or mortgage payments, utilities, transportation, maintenance, food, clothing, insurance premiums, taxes, installment payments, medical expenses, support expenses - and "non-essential" or discretionary expenses, such as dining out, entertainment, vacations, charitable contributions, and gifts.

Finally, review your potential sources of retirement income, which may include Social Security, a pension, withdrawals from retirement plans and savings accounts, annuity income, rental real estate income, and earned income from a part-time job.

All your living expenses, essential and discretionary, should be less than your after-tax income; otherwise, you run the risk of going into debt and/or outliving your assets. At the very least, you should have enough after-tax income to cover your essential expenses. The traditional rule of thumb is to have a retirement plan that replaces 80% of your pre-retirement income, but this is just a general rule. The needs and desires of each retired individual or couple is different. Those who plan to travel or undertake costly hobbies might need a higher percentage in retirement, but for many people, the amount needed is closer to 60%. In addition, income needs often decline over time; as a person ages, they usually travel less, dine out less, etc. On the flip side, as people age, their medical expenses often increase over time. You can often lower your living expenses by downsizing your home and moving to a less expensive area. Also, by taking better care of your health, as discussed in the first part of this book, you could potentially reduce your healthcare costs.

Paying Off Debt

When assessing your finances, you must consider the amount and type of debt that you have, if any. If you are carrying a mortgage or credit card debt into retirement, and you have money sitting in a low interest account, such as a bank savings account, it is probably a good idea to use that money to pay off your higher-interest debt. After all, paying off debt gives you an equivalent guaranteed rate of return. For example, if you carry a credit card balance with an interest rate of 12%, and your bank is paying you 2% interest on a CD, by paying off the debt with the CD money, you have given yourself an equivalent 10% net guaranteed rate of return (12% - 2% = 10%.) Note: there may be fees for cashing in a CD before maturity. Once you retire, you should use credit cards only if you plan to pay the entire balance each statement period, so you won't accrue interest. (Paying off your credit card balance every month is a good habit to start well before retirement.) Although not as crucial, if you are carrying a mortgage into retirement, and it is not possible to earn at least the equivalent interest in a risk-free investment, you might also consider paying off the mortgage if you have the cash to do so. On the other hand, if you are buying a car, and you are offered an extremely low interest rate to finance the car, such as 0-1%, then it probably makes sense to finance the car, as opposed to taking the money out of the bank and buying it outright. A good website to compare interest rates on CDs, savings accounts, mortgage rates, and car loan rates is https://www.bankrate.com/.

Supporting Adult Children

When you are employed and have a steady paycheck, you might be in a good position to help your adult children with expenses, provide regular cash gifts, or a free place to live. But when you retire, each dollar you give to or spend on your children is one less dollar you will have to support yourself throughout retirement, which could last a long time. Although cutting off your children from financial support may be difficult, it does not have to be cold turkey. As your retirement nears, you could explain that you will be gradually cutting back on gifts and money for their expenses, because, once retired, you will be living on a fixed income. You could further explain that, if you spend too much money in retirement, you could become a financial burden to them in the future. They should understand and appreciate the point.

Sources of Retirement Income

While we touched upon various sources of retirement income in Chapters 3 and 5, we will now discuss those sources in more detail.

Social Security

Among other things, Social Security is designed to provide financial support to retired and disabled people to cover essential living expenses. Many people are concerned about the future of Social Security. According to a Social Security consumer survey, "72% of future retirees worry that Social Security will run out of funding in their lifetimes."[2] But, "The latest Board of Trustees report estimates benefits will remain fully payable until at least 2034, with 79% of benefits payable through 2091, and 74% of benefits payable thereafter."[3] So, while the U.S. Government may eventually need to make some changes to address Social Security's long-term funding shortfalls (which might include a delayed retirement age, higher taxes, and means testing), a large portion of the future Social Security benefits appears to be secure. Alarmingly, many future retirees don't fully understand their Social Security benefits, often believing incorrectly that they are eligible for full benefits at an age earlier than their actual eligible age. Some also expect to receive an average of $1,805/month in benefits, when the current average payment of $1,408/month is much lower.[4] These misconceptions can pose a real challenge, especially for those people for whom Social Security will be their primary or only source of retirement income. If you fall in this category of people, it is vitally important to determine your potential Social Security benefits well in advance of retirement, as it might be a crucial part of your overall income.

In retirement, Social Security offers the following benefits:

- Lifetime retirement income
- Payments that are indexed for inflation
- Spousal and survivor benefits
- Preferential tax treatment

Not only can Social Security help fill financial gaps by covering basic retirement expenses, you can potentially increase your benefits by delaying your withdrawal of benefits to a later age, and by maximizing survivor benefits. The payment of full Social Security benefits starts for most people at ages 66 or 67. If you delay filing for benefits even later, you will receive a higher percentage of benefits for every year you delay, up to age 70. While you may file for benefits as early as age 62, you will receive a reduced monthly benefit. For example, for a person with a full retirement age of 66, filing at age 62 would result in a 25% permanent reduction of benefits, while filing at age 70 would result in a 32% permanent increase of benefits (8% increase for each year delayed). For a person with a full retirement age of 67, filing at age 62 would result in a 30% permanent reduction of benefits for filing, filing at age 70 would result in a 24% permanent increase of benefits (8% increase for each year delayed). There is a break-even point, typically between 12 to 15 years from the start of Social Security benefits, at which collecting higher benefits over a shorter period of time (delaying Social Security benefits to full retirement age or longer) is more beneficial than collecting smaller benefits over a longer period of time (starting Social Security benefits at age 62). There are times when it makes sense to start receiving Social Security benefits sooner, even if at a reduced amount, such as an unexpected early retirement or poor health. But there are other things to consider when deciding when to file, such as benefits for your spouse, benefits for dependent children, your present health and life expectancy, your other sources of retirement income, and tax ramifications. Remember, in addition to benefits for your current spouse, your Social Security might also provide benefits to surviving spouses and divorced spouses.

If you are younger than 70, and have already begun collecting Social Security benefits, you are entitled to suspend payments, and start collecting again at age 70. In that scenario, your benefits would earn delayed retirement credits of 8% per year from the time you suspend benefits up until age 70. If you filed your initial claim for Social Security benefits within the past 12 months, you could withdraw your application and reapply at a future date. But keep in mind that you must repay all the benefits that you and your family members have already received. Also, be aware that you are entitled to only one withdrawal per lifetime. Because there is a lot to consider when filing for Social Security benefits, you may want to speak to your financial advisor for guidance. According to a Social Security Consumer Survey conducted by Harris Poll on behalf of the Nationwide Retirement Institute, 2017, "Those working with a financial advisor receive almost 20% more in Social Security benefits than those who do not. Yet, less than 1 in 5 people have a financial advisor who is providing them with Social Security advice."[5] You will also find pertinent information at https://www.ssa.gov/ and https://www.ssa.gov/benefits/retirement/planner/otherthings.html.

Pensions

A pension plan is a defined benefit retirement plan that requires an employer to make contributions into a pool of funds that are set aside for their employees' retirement. This pool of funds is invested to meet future obligations. Typically, at retirement, an individual with a pension plan can choose to receive a series of payments, usually paid over the course of his/her life, or they can choose a lump sum payment. The number of workers in private sector jobs who have defined benefit plans has been falling drastically over the years. From 1975 to 2005, the number of private sector workers with a defined benefit pension has dropped from 88 percent to 33 percent, and continues to drop.[6] Defined benefit pension plans often provide guaranteed lifetime income payments, but due to the high cost of maintaining this type of plan, many companies have shifted toward defined contribution plans instead. Employer contribution plans provide an accumulation benefit, but no lifetime income payments. If you are fortunate to have a pension plan, you have another layer of guaranteed lifetime income in addition to your Social Security income.

Withdrawals from Taxable Accounts

Investors seeking income from taxable accounts often choose:

- Dividend-paying equity investments (individual stocks, and mutual funds and exchange traded funds (ETFs) that invest in stocks)
- Fixed income investments (CDs, bonds, preferred stocks, and mutual funds and ETFs that invest in these investments)
- Alternative tangible investments (real estate investment trusts (REITs)

Some of these assets also have the potential for growth and growth of income, which can offset the impacts of inflation. While it makes sense to maintain an investment portfolio of these types of equities, fixed-income, and alternative assets, these assets do carry investment risk (discussed further in Chapter 10). For instance, during a bear market (downward market trend), dividend-paying equities might experience loss of principal and the corporations may have to reduce or eliminate their dividends altogether, as some companies did during the significant market downturn in 2008-2009 and again in 2020. In addition, fixed income investments and alternative investments might also lose value and reduce or eliminate their interest payments.

Withdrawals from Retirement Accounts

A major source of income for many retirees is withdrawals from their retirement accounts, including IRAs and qualified retirement plans, such as 401(k), profit sharing plans, 403(b), 457(b), SEP-IRAs and SIMPLE IRAs. In the recent past, an annual withdrawal rate of 4%, adjusted for inflation, was considered a sustainable withdrawal rate. But today, when you factor in the volatility of the stock market, persistently low interest rates, fees, and longevity (people are living longer on average), the safer, sustaining withdrawal rate appears to be less than 2%.[7] According to an article by Dr. Wade Phau and Wade Dokken, both well known in the financial industry, "Recent research that Dr. Pfau and I have conducted finds that investors retiring as of January 1, 2015, who pursue a traditional 4% withdrawal rate from their savings to fund retirement have a more than 50% chance of outliving their savings."[8] Furthermore, although on average, stock market returns over a period of 30-40 years have been high, negative returns occurring early in retirement can be detrimental to the portfolio, as income is withdrawn. This is known as "Sequence of Return Risk," which will be discussed in detail in Chapter 9. If you factor in that Required Minimum Distributions (RMDs) require a high withdrawal rate (see table below), it is very possible to outlive your IRA or other qualified retirement plan, especially if that account is supporting two people.

Sample of Current RMD Rate Factors/Withdrawal Percentages, at Five-Year Intervals

Age	Rate Factor	Withdrawal Percentage
70	27.4	3.65%
75	22.9	4.37%
80	18.7	5.35%
85	14.8	6.76%
90	11.4	8.77%

As previously discussed, RMDs require you to take distributions from your traditional IRAs and qualified retirement plans at age 72, even if you don't need the income at that time. (As a reminder, the RMD age was recently changed from age 70 ½ to age 72 for individuals who turn age 70 ½ in 2020.) Again, RMDs must be taken by the end of each calendar year, except for the first RMD, which can be deferred until April 1 of the following calendar year. In addition, if you defer your initial RMD to the next calendar year, you must take two RMDs that following year. The penalty for not taking the RMD is 50% of the required RMD amount that should have been taken and you would still be required to take the missed RMD.

Annuity Income

The dual impact of longevity risk and sequence of return risk creates the real possibility that withdrawals from an investment portfolio might not support your desired lifestyle over the entire period of your retirement. In retirement, we face two foundational unknowns: our individual life expectancy, and the future returns of the stock and bond markets. A safeguard against these risks can be to pool investments into annuities, thereby minimizing the risks of fluctuating markets and the risk of running out of money.

Annuities can provide income for a specified period, or for the lifetime of the annuitant. Depending on the type of annuity, this income can be fixed or variable, and may provide guaranteed lifetime income for one or two people. In addition to Social Security benefits and pensions, annuities provide a supplemental guaranteed income stream. Annuities will be discussed in greater detail in Chapter 12.

Rental Real Estate Income

Real estate is another potential income source in retirement. However, investment properties should provide a steady positive cash flow, and not become a drain on your retirement income and assets. Financing an investment property generally requires a down payment of 20% or more. Paying cash for real estate ties up money that could otherwise be invested into interest or dividend-producing investments. When purchasing investment properties, it is prudent to also set aside enough money to cover taxes, insurance, and the mortgage (for properties that are financed) for times of vacancy and for unexpected repairs that could occur at any time. Again, setting aside extra cash to cover these costs ties up money that could be otherwise invested. The tax benefits of investment properties can be beneficial, but complex, so it is wise to seek the advice of a good tax professional in advance. When shopping for an investment property, be sure to work with an experienced and trusted realtor. Lastly, keep in mind that being a landlord can become a part-time job, so be sure you understand the ins and outs before you venture into rental real estate.[9]

Reverse Mortgages

A reverse mortgage is a type of loan that allows homeowners, age 62 or older, to borrow from the equity in their home. This money can be borrowed as a lump sum, fixed monthly payments, or line of credit, and the loan is not due until the borrower moves, sells the house, or dies. Reverse mortgages were created to help retirees with limited income use the equity in their homes to cover basic living expenses, but the money can be used for anything. Borrowers must remain current on property taxes, homeowner's insurance, and association dues (if applicable). For more information, please visit: https://www.reversemortgage.org/.

Earned Income from a Part-Time Job

It is not uncommon for people to continue to work well into their 60's, 70's or even 80's. "According to the U.S. Bureau of Labor Statistics, between 1977 and 2007, the employment of workers age 65 and older rose by 101 percent. Though the number of employed people age 76 and older is relatively small, this group increased by 172 percent."[10] Some workers are forced to retire because of downsizing, poor health, or to care for a loved one, but increasingly, older Americans are choosing to stay at their jobs or start new ones. Employment income can reduce or delay withdrawals from investment accounts, giving those accounts more time to grow. Also, working keeps people mentally sharp, and gives them a sense of purpose.

As you can see, there are many potential sources of retirement income. Some provide steady, guaranteed lifetime income, such as Social Security, pensions, and annuity income (annuities can also reduce two big retirement risks, longevity risk and sequence of return risk, discussed in more detail in Chapter 9).

CHAPTER 8: WITHDRAWAL RISK

During retirement, a retiree transitions from earning and saving money to drawing income from the money they have accumulated and invested. Developing a plan to spend down assets can be particularly challenging, especially since you don't know how long you will live. Determining the appropriate withdrawal rate includes many factors, such as your income needs, inflation, asset allocation, and longevity or life expectancy. When determining appropriate withdrawal rates for your investments, also consider withdrawal risk, which is the risk of spending down assets too aggressively to meet your expenses. If the withdrawal rate is too high, you run the risk of depleting your assets and running out of income during your lifetime. As discussed in the previous chapter, at one point, a 4% withdrawal rate from investments was once considered a "safe" rate, but considering the volatility of the stock market, low interest rates, investment fees, and the fact that people are living longer, it now appears a safe withdrawal rate is closer to 2%. Of course, during an extended bull market, an appropriate withdrawal rate might be higher, but there is no way of predicting how the stock market will perform. To manage risk, you will want to assess your situation annually; you may want to adjust your withdrawal rate up or down, depending on the previous year's portfolio returns. If you face lower or negative returns early on in retirement, you will most likely need to reduce your withdrawal amounts; higher returns early on may allow you to increase your withdrawal amounts. A capable financial advisor can help you make these calculations.

I have worked with clients who, despite my advice that their withdrawal rate was unsustainable, continued to take high withdrawals from their investments. Sadly, but not surprisingly, those clients eventually ran out of money. A high withdrawal rate puts an investor in the difficult position of having to invest their money in higher yielding, but riskier investments than would otherwise be required if they were taking a lower withdrawal rate. If a high withdrawal rate is necessary to cover one's living expenses, one solution is to invest in an annuity, which can guarantee lifetime income and may offer a higher withdrawal rate than other alternatives. Annuities will be discussed in more detail in Chapter 12.

CHAPTER 9:
SEQUENCE OF RETURN RISK

Sequence of return risk, or sequence risk, is the danger that the timing of retirement investment withdrawals will negatively impact the anticipated long-term return on the investor's portfolio. Sequence risk involves the order in which investment returns occur, and the impact it will have on your money. During the accumulation period of your investments, when you are normally still contributing and not taking any withdrawals from your investment portfolio, the sequence of returns makes little difference. But during the distribution period, when you are no longer contributing, and are taking withdrawals from your investment portfolio, sequence of returns can make a huge difference.

Accumulation Phase

The following example shows two portfolios in the accumulation stage: Portfolio A and Portfolio B, each with a starting value of $100,000. What happens when the sequence of annual returns is reversed? In portfolio A, there are 3 years of negative returns on investment at the beginning of the accumulation stage, while in portfolio B, there are 3 years of negative returns at the end of the accumulation stage. As you can see, the average annual returns for both portfolios is 8%, and the ending values are exactly the same, $684,848.

Accumulation Phase Example

The sequence of returns for portfolio A and B have been reversed, with no withdrawals taken.

	Portfolio A	Portfolio B
Starting Value:	$100,000	$100,000
Average Rate of Return:	8%	8%
Withdrawals:	None	None
Value at Age 65:	$684,848	$684,848

Age	Annual Return Portfolio A	Year-end Value Portfolio A	Annual Return Portfolio B	Year-End Value Portfolio B
Start		$100,000		$100,000
41	-12%	$87,695	29%	$129,491
42	-21%	$69,426	18%	$152,281
43	-14%	$59,707	25%	$189,590
44	22%	$72,984	-6%	$178,404
45	10%	$80,136	15%	$204,272
46	4%	$83,595	8%	$221,183
47	11%	$92,707	27%	$281,124
48	3%	$95,210	-2%	$274,939
49	-3%	$92,155	15%	$315,355
50	21%	$111,507	19%	$375,272
51	17%	$130,129	33%	$498,737
52	5%	$137,026	11%	$554,097
53	-10%	$123,597	-10%	$499,795
54	11%	$137,316	5%	$526,284
55	33%	$182,493	17%	$614,174
56	19%	$217,167	21%	$743,150
57	15%	$249,091	-3%	$719,305
58	-2%	$243,611	3%	$738,726
59	27%	$309,629	11%	$819,247
60	8%	$335,262	4%	$854,602
61	15%	$383,875	10%	$938,354
62	-6%	$361,226	22%	$1,147,022
63	25%	$449,727	-14%	$986,439
64	18%	$528,878	-21%	$780,941
65	29%	$684,848	-12%	$684,848
	Average: 8%	$684,848	Average: 8%	$684,848

Distribution Phase

During the distribution phase, however, the relationship between your rate of withdrawal and the sequence of returns can have a dramatic impact on your investment portfolio's ability to last throughout your retirement. In the following example, Portfolio A and Portfolio B both have a starting value of $684,848 (the ending value in the previous example). In this scenario, 5% of the first-year value is taken as a withdrawal, adjusted thereafter for inflation. Now what happens when the sequence of annual returns is once again reversed? In portfolio A, there are 3 years of negative returns at the beginning of the distribution stage, while in portfolio B, there are 3 years of negative returns at the end of the distribution stage. The average annual rate of return remains 8% in both portfolios. As you can see, in Portfolio A, the investor ran out of money at age 82, while in portfolio B, the investor ended up with a lot more money than they had at the outset. Portfolio A could not recover from the early losses because distributions were taken when large portfolio losses occurred.

Distribution Phase Example

The sequence of returns for portfolio A and B have been reversed. Both portfolios are taking withdrawals of 5% of the starting value, adjusted annually for inflation.

	Portfolio A	Portfolio B
Starting Value:	$648,848	$648,848
Average Rate of Return:	8%	8%
Annual Withdrawals:	5%*	5%*
Value at Age 90:	$0	$2,622,984

*Annual Withdrawals: 5% of first year value adjusted annually for inflation.

Age	Annual Return Portfolio A	Year-end Value Portfolio A	Annual Return Portfolio B	Year-End Value Portfolio B
65		$648,848		$648,848
66	-12%	$566,337	29%	$852,571
67	-21%	$413,086	18%	$967,355
68	-14%	$318,927	25%	$1,168,029
69	22%	$352,432	-6%	$1,061,698
70	10%	$348,432	15%	$1,177,105
71	4%	$323,772	8%	$1,234,855
72	11%	$318,176	27%	$1,528,614
73	3%	$284,653	-2%	$1,452,871
74	-3%	$232,143	15%	$1,623,066
75	21%	$236,215	19%	$1,886,771
76	17%	$229,644	33%	$2,461,500
77	5%	$194,417	11%	$2,687,327
78	-10%	$126,543	-10%	$2,375,148
79	11%	$90,304	5%	$2,450,746
80	33%	$68,219	17%	$2,808,226
81	19%	$27,833	21%	$3,344,606
82	15%	$0	-3%	$3,182,338
83	-2%	$0	3%	$3,211,664
84	27%	$0	11%	$3,503,440
85	8%	$0	4%	$3,594,592
86	15%	$0	10%	$3,885,017
87	-6%	$0	22%	$4,685,257
88	25%	$0	-14%	$3,963,710
89	18%	$0	-21%	$3,070,398
90	29%	$0	-12%	$2,622,984
	Average: 8%	$0	Average: 8%	$2,622,984

Since nobody can predict when the stock market will have good years and bad years, sequence of return risk can be a major risk in retirement. This is especially true for those that retire at the end of a bull market. "In an increasingly volatile world, planning for such a potential scenario and structuring a retirement income portfolio to guard against such a risk seems both prudent and realistic. It also supports the case for utilizing some type of annuity as insurance against that risk."[1] Annuities will be discussed in more detail in Chapter 12.

CHAPTER 10: INVESTMENT RISK

In simple terms, investment risk is the probability or likelihood of losing money on a particular investment. Some of the risks that affect investors are:

- **Market Risk:** the possibility of losing money in the securities markets, which include equities, fixed income, and derivatives. Equity securities include individual stocks, mutual funds and exchange traded funds (ETFs) that invest in stocks. Fixed income securities include individual bonds, mutual funds and ETFs that invest in bonds. Derivative securities include various forms of options contracts. Market risk can occur because of changes in interest rates, political uncertainty, economic recessions, terrorist attacks and pandemics.

- **Investment Concentration Risk:** the risk of having a large portion of your assets in one or a limited amount of investments. For example, owning stocks or bonds in only one company could expose you to large losses upon adverse news of the company.

- **Interest-Rate Risk:** the risk of being locked into a low interest rate in a period when interest rates are rising. Interest rate changes can affect fixed income investment prices. As interest rates increase, the value of many types of fixed income investments decrease.

- **Credit Risk:** the risk of default on a debt because the borrower is unable to make required payments. The risk includes the loss of principal and interest.

- **Call Risk/Reinvestment Risk:** the risk that your investment will be called/sold prior to maturity, and you are unable to reinvest cash flows at a rate equal to that investment.

- **Inflation Risk:** the risk that the cash flows from an investment will be worth less in the future due to the impact of inflation. This is also known as purchasing power risk.

In addition to the above risks, the following factors should be considered when constructing an investment portfolio:

- Your entire financial picture, including your income and expenses, your assets and liabilities, and the size of your emergency fund
- Your investment goals and objectives
- Your time horizon
- Your liquidity needs
- Your risk tolerance

You can construct a portfolio on your own, or with the help of a financial advisor.

Many of the risks listed above can be mitigated by diversification. A definition of diversification is "a risk management strategy that mixes a wide variety of investments within a portfolio. The rationale behind this technique is that a portfolio constructed of different kinds of assets will, on average, yield higher long-term returns and lower the risk of any individual holding or security."[1] But keep in mind that, although risk can be reduced by diversification, it cannot be eliminated. Let's discuss how diversification can help to reduce the risks discussed earlier.

Market Risk

By constructing a portfolio of different asset classes, including stocks, bonds, cash, and "hard or tangible assets" like real estate and commodities, you reduce the risk that all assets will decrease in value at the same time. This is known as asset allocation. "The decision of how much goes into each category (stocks, bonds, or cash, for example) has proven to be more significant than the selection of the specific stock, fund, real estate, or other investment and may account for as much as 80 percent of the overall return on the portfolio."[2] The idea of diversification is that, if you hold investments with negative correlations - meaning that one investment may increase in value while another decreases in value - this balancing should theoretically reduce your risk and smooth out your returns. For example, stocks and bonds don't always move in the same direction, making bonds a good diversification vehicle against stock market risk.

Market Timing vs. Buy and Hold

You could attempt to reduce or eliminate market risk by trying to time the market, which is a strategy of buying low and selling high. The idea behind this principle is to buy a security or a basket of securities when it is low and sell it when it is high (buy low, sell high). But how do you know when an investment (or the market) has reached its high and its low? Simple answer - you don't. It is all speculation and luck. While you might get lucky on occasion, most of the time, you **will** be wrong.

Since market timing very seldomly works, many investors simply buy and hold for the long term, with the belief and understanding that markets go up over time. By constructing a portfolio mix of investments with lower correlations (i.e., stocks and bonds), you can potentially reduce losses when the stock market drops. For example, during a market downturn, a portfolio with a mix of stocks, bonds, and cash, should drop less than a portfolio with 100% stocks. On the other hand, in a rising stock market, a diversified portfolio might lag in comparison to the returns of a portfolio comprised of 100% stocks. One way to measure the risk of an investment or an investment portfolio is by something called "beta", which is a measurement of the investment's or portfolio's sensitivity to market risk. The S&P 500®, as a broad measurement of the stock market, has a beta of 1. This means that an investment asset or portfolio with a beta below 1 would indicate it is less volatile than the market. So for instance, during a market downturn, an asset or portfolio with a beta of .5 should drop about half as much as the S&P 500®, and increase about half as much as the S&P 500® when the stock market rises. On the other hand, an investment or portfolio with a beta of 2 would indicate more volatility. During a market downturn, an asset with a beta of 2 should drop about twice as much as the S&P 500® and increase about twice as much as the S&P 500® when the stock market rises. The problem with the buy and hold strategy is that it takes a great deal of faith and discipline to not sell your investments when your portfolio value is rapidly dropping in value. When markets are tumbling, many investors get emotional and sell their investments because they fear losing most or all their investments. But this is often the worst possible time to sell investments. Back in 2008, I was working with a client who wanted to sell when the markets were plummeting. His exact words were, "I want to stop the bleeding." I asked him if he needed the money that day, and when he said no, I asked, "so why sell now"? I suggested that he wait it out and sell when the markets eventually rebounded. He took my advice and eventually recouped his losses.

Investment Concentration Risk

Diversification can greatly reduce investment concentration risk, which is the risk of greater losses occurring from holding a large portion of your portfolio's assets in one investment or asset class. In that situation, a drop in value of a concentrated security might cause a more significant loss in a portfolio's value than if the portfolio were more diversified. For example, an employee who accumulates a large amount of company stock puts himself/herself at greater risk if the company performs poorly. In addition to losing value in the company stock, the employee might also lose his/her job; and if the company were to go bankrupt, the employee could lose everything. There are many real-life examples of this, such as Enron, Lehman Brothers, and General Motors. Anyone who had a large concentration of stock in these companies may have been wiped out. On the other hand, investing in a broad index, such as the S&P 500®, spreads your investments over 500 companies, and significantly reduces your investment concentration risk. Even if one or two companies in the S&P 500® were to go bankrupt, your losses would be limited, and you would not lose your entire investment.

Again, while diversification can reduce risk, it does not eliminate it altogether. Moreover, it is possible to overdiversify, and reduce the upside potential of your portfolio. Holding too many investments can spread your portfolio so thin that any movement upward in one or two holdings might not materially impact your returns. The way to truly diversify your portfolio is to buy stocks that are diversified in size, industry, sector, country, etc. This can be done through individual stocks, mutual funds, or ETFs. Keep in mind, if you own a large concentrated position of XYZ stock in a qualified retirement account or an IRA, you can sell it and diversify without any tax consequences. However, if you own the same concentrated position of XYZ stock in a taxable account, and there is a low-cost basis, selling your shares would incur a large capital gains tax. If selling a concentrated position in stocks would incur a large capital gain, there are two approaches to managing concentrated stock risk, Exchange Funds and Stock Protection Funds.

Exchange Funds

In an exchange fund, individual investors, each with concentrated stock positions in different companies, contribute shares of their stocks into one pool, in exchange for an ownership interest in the entire pool's portfolio. In a (simplified) nutshell, after seven years, each investor receives a diverse basket of individual stocks. This strategy provides investors an easy way to diversify their concentrated stock positions while deferring capital gains tax.

Stock Protection Funds

In a stock protection fund, individual investors, each with concentrated stock positions in different companies, contribute a modest amount of cash into a fund in exchange for an ownership interest in the fund. The cash position is invested conservatively in U.S. bonds for the term of the fund (usually five years). When the fund matures, the cash is used to partially or totally reimburse investors whose stocks have lost money, and any excess cash is returned to shareholders. This strategy allows investors to remain invested in concentrated stock positions while reducing investment concentration risk.

To learn more about these two strategies, please visit: https://www.wealthmanagement.com/alternative-investments/consider-stock-protection-funds-de-risking-concentrated-positions.

Interest Rate Risk

Interest rate risk, which specifically affects bonds and other fixed-income investments, such as preferred stocks, is the risk that changes in interest rates might reduce the value of those fixed-income investments. When interest rates rise, the market value of most bonds or bond funds tends to drop. Conversely, when interest rates fall, the market value of most bonds or bond funds tends to increase. The reason for this can be explained in the following examples. Let's say you bought a $1,000 10-year bond with a coupon interest rate of 2%, and then interest rates rise to 3%. Now, if you wanted to sell your bond before its maturity date, the bond would sell at a discounted rate (below $1,000), because a new, higher-interest bond (3%) is available for $1,000. In other words, your bond is no longer appealing for $1,000, because the same money begets a higher interest bond. The converse is also true. Using the same cost/coupon rate of the previous example, if interest rates were to drop to 1%, then your bond would likely sell at a premium.

The interest sensitivity of a fixed-income asset is an assessment of how much the price is likely to fluctuate with an upward or downward movement of interest rates. More sensitive assets have greater price fluctuations than less sensitive assets. One way to measure the interest sensitivity of a bond or bond fund is by its duration period, which is indicated in years. The longer the duration, the more sensitive the bond or bond fund will be to changes in interest rates. So, if interest rates were to increase by 1%, then the price of a bond fund with a duration of 5 years would be expected to decrease by 5%. Conversely, if interest rates were to decrease by 1%, then the bond fund's price would be expected to increase by 5%. Note that holding an individual bond to maturity eliminates the bond's interest rate risk, as the par or face value of the bond will be paid. Unlike individual bonds, bond *funds* do not have a maturity date, so they always carry some interest rate risk.

There are certain bonds or bond funds, called Bank Loans, or Senior Floating Rate bonds, that don't have fixed interest rates. Instead, these bonds/bond funds have "floating" or variable interest rates, which means that the interest rate paid on the bond changes over time, based on a particular reference rate, such as the London Interbank Offered Rate (LIBOR) or the Federal Funds rate. These bonds are less interest rate sensitive than traditional bonds, but they usually carry higher credit risk, discussed below.

Credit Risk

Bonds and other fixed-income investments can also carry credit risk, also known as default risk. It is the risk that the bond issuer will default on its obligations, resulting in the bond holder not getting paid principal and interest. Some bonds are riskier than others. For example, U.S. Treasury bonds are generally thought of as free from default risk, while lower-rated bonds or junk bonds have a higher risk of default. There are rating organizations, such as Moody's, Standard & Poor's, and Fitch, that rate the credit risk of bonds. These ratings range from AAA, the highest rating, to D, the worst rating (which is assigned to bonds that are already in default). Because a lower-rated bond has a greater default risk, it generally pays a higher interest rate than a higher-rated bond to compensate for the greater default risk.

Call Risk/Reinvestment Risk

Call risk is yet another risk of bonds and other fixed-income investments. If the bond is callable, meaning it may be redeemed by the issuer before its maturity date, the issuer could call the bond when interest rates drop. Doing so allows the issuer to issue new bonds at lower rates, thus saving the issuer money. When a bond is called, the bond principal is paid to the investor, who now needs to find a suitable replacement. Given that interest rates have fallen, finding a replacement is often difficult to do. This is known as reinvestment risk. Reinvestment risk is most common with bond investments, but any investment that generates cash flow exposes the investor to this type of risk.

Reducing Bond Risks (Interest Rate Risk, Credit Risk and Call Risk/ Reinvestment Risk)

Interest rate risk and credit risk can be reduced by investing in a diversified bond fund or ETF that holds many bonds with different degrees of interest rate risk and credit risk. The bond fund's duration will convey the fund's overall interest rate risk, and the average bond rating will convey its overall credit risk. Many bond funds hold 1,000 bond issues or more, greatly reducing credit risk. Call risk can be eliminated simply by buying bonds that are not callable.

Inflation Risk

Perhaps the greatest risk to your investment portfolio and your future income is inflation risk. Inflation will decrease your purchasing power over time. For some people, this could mean giving up some of life's luxuries, but for others, this could mean having to make hard choices, such as cutting down on some necessities, or going back to work. Retirees are especially susceptible to inflation, because the cost of goods and services purchased by retirees, such as healthcare and long-term care, tends to increase faster than the general inflation rate. Bonds and low interest-bearing accounts, such as money market accounts and CDs, are usually poor hedges against inflation. Stocks, real estate, and other tangible assets are generally a good hedge against inflation. If a retiree were to invest $1,000,000 in a 30-year treasury bond paying 2% interest, they would receive $20,000 a year of safe, steady, dependable income. The retiree might be able to sleep at night knowing that their principal and interest are safe, but what they might not notice right away is that their income is not keeping pace with inflation. While the cost of living increases each year, their income remains fixed at $20,000, so their purchasing power decreases over time. At 3% average inflation, the purchasing power of their income will be cut in half in 24 years (Rule of 72: 72 divided by 3 equals 24). At 4% average inflation, the purchasing power of their income will be cut in half in 18 years (72 divided by 4 equals 18).

Ways to Reduce Inflation Risk

One way to reduce inflation risk is to purchase Treasury Inflation-Protected Securities (TIPS), which adjust their principal upon changes in the consumer price index (CPI), giving the investor a real inflation-adjusted return on their investment. Interest on TIPS is paid every six months and can vary, since the rate is applied to the adjusted principal of the bond. If the principal increases over time due to inflation, the interest rate is applied to that higher principal amount, providing the investor with higher income. The converse is also true. If deflation occurs, the investor will receive a lower income. Although TIPS can be a hedge against inflation, they tend to pay lower interest than similar fixed income investments, so they may be less advantageous for investors seeking higher income. If inflation does not materialize while the TIPS are held, then the benefits of owning them disappear.[3]

Other ways to reduce inflation risk include:

- Avoid holding a high concentration of long-term bonds that pay a fixed coupon rate.

- Own a diversified mix of stocks, real estate, or real estate investment trusts (REITs), and other tangible assets in your investment portfolio.

- Postpone taking Social Security income. Since Social Security has annual cost of living adjustments, the longer you wait to collect (up to age 70), the higher your Social Security payments (and future cost of living adjustments) will be.

- Purchase an annuity that has the potential to pay a rising income.

- Decrease your living expenses.

As you can see, there are many risks associated with investing. While these risks can never be entirely eliminated, they can be reduced with some of the strategies discussed in this chapter. It is important to understand these risks and how they can destroy your wealth. A financial advisor can be a valuable resource in identifying these risks and offering potential solutions to reduce these risks.

CHAPTER 11:
INVESTOR BEHAVIOR

"Do people act rationally when making decisions about their investments? Most economic and financial theory is based on the premise that people do act logically and consider all available information in the decision-making process. However, a surprising amount of evidence exists indicating that human beings show repeated patterns of inconsistency, irrationality, and incompetence when faced with decisions or choices that deal with uncertainty."[1] There are several real-world examples of this, including:

- The Dutch Tulip Bubble of the 1630s
- The South Sea Bubble of 1720
- Japan's Real Estate and Stock Market Bubble of 1990
- The Dot-Com Bubble of 2000-2002
- The U.S. Housing and Credit Bubble of 2008

Investors have always been, and will continue to be, influenced by their emotions. "As investors, we have to recognize that our individual emotional behavior can be our own worst enemy."[2] "As long as human emotions are a factor in financial decision making, we are likely to repeat the lessons of the past and experience periods of frenzied euphoria followed by times of despair and depression."[3] Behavioral finance attempts to understand how emotions influence the decision-making process of investors. "One of the pioneers of behavioral finance was the late Amos Tversky, professor of psychology at Stanford University. Tversky found that individuals are much more distressed by prospective losses than they are happy with equivalent gains. Faced with a sure gain, many investors become risk averse, but faced with a sure loss, investors become risk takers."[4] Many investors tend to be hesitant to sell investments that have dropped in value, even if there is a good reason to sell. By not selling, they are unwilling to realize their losses and their mistakes. They cling onto the belief that a loss is not a loss until it is realized. Some investors take on even more risk by investing additional capital in a down-trending investment to "average down" their purchase cost. This behavior often leads to more losses. On the other hand, investors are also often unwilling to sell investments that have gone up in value, in the fear of missing out on further gains. These indecisions often leave investors paralyzed in their decision making. Additionally, some investors tend to cope with portfolio losses by ignoring them. When markets are doing well, investors enjoy reviewing their statements, but when markets are performing poorly, investors tend to ignore their statements.

Confirmation Bias

"Confirmation bias is the tendency to search for, interpret, favor, and recall information in a way that confirms one's preexisting beliefs or hypotheses. People display this bias when they gather or remember information selectively, or when they interpret it in a biased way. The effect is stronger for desired outcomes, emotionally charged issues, and for deeply entrenched beliefs."[5] In other words, people tend to hear what they want to hear. For example, when investors believe that the stock market or an individual stock will continue to increase or decrease in value, they tend to seek out information that confirms their beliefs and ignore any information that contradicts it.

Recency Bias

People tend to recall and emphasize recent events and observations, more so than recalling those that occurred in the past. When the stock market is rising, investors tend to believe it will continue to rise, so they tend to buy stocks. On the other hand, when the stock market is dropping, investors tend to believe it will continue to fall, so they tend to sell stocks. This can lead markets to soar upward or plunge downward in an exaggerated way. In the late 1990s and early in 2000, investors were overconfident that the stock market would continue to rise, and they continued to pile into stocks, even though the stock market, particularly the tech heavy NASDAQ market, was extremely overvalued at the time. This confidence led to more buying and more speculation, until the stock market ultimately crashed. Contrarily, during "The Great Recession" of 2008-2009, investors feared that the stock market would continue to sell off, and they continued selling stocks until the market bottomed out in March of 2009. Even after the market started moving upwards, investors sat on the sidelines, waiting for confirmation that things had gotten better.

According to Robert Shiller, a Yale University economist, human behavior is what drives stock prices. Shiller opines further that the "Efficient-Market Theory" - the idea that financial prices accurately reflect all public information at all times, or in other words, that stocks are correctly priced all the time - is completely wrong. Schiller's belief appears to have support, as the stock market often fluctuates wildly up or down based on breaking global news. "Logically, each publicly traded company is producing the same product and service as it was just minutes before the news, but the reaction of the investor is irrationally euphoric or catastrophically morose. Internet technology has made it too convenient for investors to make rash decisions based upon their emotional reactions."[6]

Information Overload

In the distant past, before the days of the internet, investors would receive and review their account statements each quarter, and that was it. They would look up stock and mutual fund prices in the next day's newspaper. There was much less trading, and investors tended to hold their investments for long periods of time. But then came the internet and news stations feverishly covering the markets, minute by minute, giving investors instant information and the ability to view and trade their accounts daily, including their 401k plans. This intensity and bombardment of investment information exploded in the late 1990s and early 2000, when some investors quit their day jobs to become "day traders"; this did not end well for many people. This information overload has led to more market volatility than I can remember. Negative news attracts more viewers, and news stations understand this. People tune in in droves when the stock market is tumbling, and less so when the stock market is stable or rising.

Herd Mentality Bias

Herd mentality bias is the tendency of an investor to behave like other investors, such as buying the same or similar investments based solely on the fact that others (especially family/friends, colleagues, acquaintances) are buying those investments. It's the age-old fear of missing out. Herd mentality is a significant driver of asset bubbles in the financial markets. For example, in the late 1990s and early 2000, investors were buying anything that had a "dot com" attached to it, regardless of whether the company was profitable or not. These same investors ended up selling their positions when those stocks got crushed. A similar bubble happened in the years leading up to 2008, when investors were speculating on real estate, and banks were happy to lend to anyone, regardless of their credit score. Wall Street was more than happy to package these speculative loans into investments, which were then given an investment grade rating by the rating agencies. We all know how it ended. The movie, "The Big Short" is a great reminder of this herd-mentality-driven speculation and greed.

Investor behavior often affects an individual's investment performance. The average investor has poor timing, and tends to buy high, chasing returns, and sell low, when markets become volatile. This behavior can be very costly. For example, in 2018, the S&P 500® lost 4.4% for the year. The average investor, on the other hand, lost 9.4%.[7] Stock mutual fund investors underperformed the S&P 500® by an average of 5.88% yearly over 30 years, ending 12/31/2018.[8] Over the long-term, an investor's underperformance can cost them a great deal of money. Investors who work with financial advisors tend to do better than those who don't. In 2001, Vanguard funds, a well-recognized investment management company, released a study, "Advisor's Alpha". "This study estimates that clients who work with a good financial advisor will receive on average a 3% increase in the value of their portfolios each year. Of course, this increase does not come in a linear, orderly fashion. The majority of this increase will come during periods of heightened greed and fear in the markets when advisors can step in and help their clients maintain an even keel and keep their long-term objectives in sight. These studies ultimately show that financial advisors truly earn their fees by acting as behavioral coaches rather than money managers."[9] In addition to helping their clients manage their emotions during market downturns, financial advisors can also help their clients plan for retirement and other financial goals.

CHAPTER 12:
FINANCIAL RISK MANAGEMENT STRATEGIES

As discussed in the previous chapters, there are many types of financial risk faced by pre-retirees and retirees, including: longevity risk; withdrawal risk; sequence of return risk; investment risk (market risk, investment concentration risk, interest-rate risk, credit risk, call risk/reinvestment risk, and inflation risk); and investor behavior. These risks can greatly affect the success of a retirement plan. While most people understand that investing in the stock market carries risk, the same people might not understand that holding money in a CD also carries risk (as previously discussed, while a CD carries no risk to principal, it does carry inflation risk). Though most investors would like to participate in stock market gains, they may not be able to handle the volatility and risk of the stock market. Investors (and their financial advisors) must have a good understanding of their risk tolerance (to determine how comfortable they are with risk), before jumping into stock market investments. While some investors can afford to ride out a bear market, not all investors can, or should. With respect to one's life savings and investments, the old saying, "hang in there" might not be the best advice for everyone, particularly those investors that are nearing retirement or have already retired.

In 2008, the S&P 500® lost roughly 37% in value, and from the peak of the market on October 9, 2007, to the bottom of the market on March 5, 2009, the S&P 500® lost roughly 56%.[1] Later in 2009, the S&P 500® rebounded, and was up over 26%. What many investors may not realize is that, when your investments lose 37%, it takes much more than a gain of 37% to make up for those losses. For example, if you had $1,000,000 invested solely in the S&P 500® at the end of 2007, your portfolio would have dropped 37%, to approximately $630,000 by the end of 2008. To recoup that $370,000 loss and get back to even, you would need a gain of close to 59%. A portfolio comprised of 60% stocks and 40% bonds during that same period would have held up much better, with losses of about 20%; a subsequent gain of 25% would get you back to even. Still, a loss of 20% is a big hit, particularly if you were taking distributions from your portfolio at the time, resulting in an even greater negative impact (see "Sequence of Return Risk" in Chapter 9).

It's interesting to note that, in a year like 2008, a mutual fund that was down less than the market was considered a success, even though it lost money. Since the 2008-2009 financial crisis, there have been several notable market corrections, including the late 2018 global market correction, and the 2020 COVID-19 market correction going on as I write this. The 2020 market correction is noteworthy because it is the fastest stock market decline from record highs, officially ending the 11-year bull market. The current markets have been extremely volatile, most likely exacerbated by negative media coverage of the pandemic, the economy, and the markets. Of course, no one wants to lose money and some investors may be willing to give up some of the upside of the stock market for less downside risk. But being too conservative can come at a price. It's important for your money to grow so that it can keep pace with inflation. Otherwise, you may end up spending down your principal too quickly and run out of money in retirement.

Mitigating Market Risk

One way to reduce stock market risk is to add bonds to the portfolio. Using the example from earlier, in 2008, a portfolio consisting of 100% stocks would have lost roughly 37% in value (as measured by the S&P 500®), while a portfolio of 60% stocks and 40% bonds would have lost roughly 20%. Bonds and stocks generally have a low correlation to one another, meaning the degree to which they move along the same lines is low. Though bonds can drop in value, since 1980, the worst calendar year performance for bonds was -2.92% (1994), as measured by the Barclays U.S. Aggregate Bond Index. This compares very favorably to stocks, whose worst calendar year performance since 1980 was -37% (2008). Between 1980 and 2018, the Barclays U.S. Aggregate Bond Index was positive for 35 out of 39 years, while the S&P 500® was positive for 31 out of 39 years.[2]

Again, bonds are not without risk. As discussed in Chapter 10, bonds are still subject to interest rate risk, credit risk, call risk/reinvestment risk, and inflation risk (see Chapter 10). Moreover, all bonds are not created equally. There are riskier bonds, such as high yield bonds, which can drop almost as much as stocks. In 2008, high yield bonds, measured by the Credit Suisse High Yield Index, lost over 26%.[3] And keep in mind that, while adding bonds to a stock portfolio will lower the portfolio's volatility, in the long-term, it may also lower the portfolio's total return. Finally, while a diversified portfolio of stocks and bonds can reduce risk, it cannot eliminate it completely. "Risk is always present because nobody can predict the future. Protecting financial assets against loss while achieving a reasonable rate of return should be the objective of both investor and adviser."[4]

Risk Management

"So, what can we do about market risk? Traditional risk management says that there are four things that we can do: avoid it, attempt to control or minimize it, retain it, or transfer it". In order to totally avoid market risk, we can simply avoid investing in the stock market. We can attempt to minimize market risk by asset allocation and diversification. We can retain market risk by directly investing in it. And lastly, we can transfer the risk to a third party. An example of risk transfer is transferring the risk of a loss to an insurance company - the premium that you pay is the cost of transferring the risk.[5] Because there is an opportunity cost of missing the higher long-term returns of the stock market, you can transfer that risk by utilizing the following investment strategies. When it comes to these strategies, the limited upside of these investments is the cost of protecting some or all of your principal. These unique investments include:

- Market-linked certificates of deposit
- Annuities
- Tactically managed mutual funds, exchange traded funds, and separately managed accounts

Market-Linked Certificates of Deposit

Though many investors are unfamiliar with market-linked certificates of deposit (MLCDs), these products have been around since 1987. The first MLCD was offered by Chase Manhattan Bank in March 1987. Initially, these CDs were purchased by institutional investors, but they have become available to individual investors, with low minimum purchase requirements. MLCDs are "structured" investment products issued by large global banks. These structured products (which include CDs and notes) are debt obligations that are linked to the market performance of their underlying equity indices, interest rates, commodities, or currency returns. Market-linked CDs offer guarantee of principal and are protected by Federal Deposit Insurance Corporation (FDIC) insurance should the issuing bank become insolvent. While Market-linked notes may offer limited or full guarantee of principal, they are not FDIC insured, so they are subject to the issuer's credit risk. The issuing bank's creditworthiness should be carefully evaluated before buying market-linked notes. Though market-linked notes tend to offer more flexibility and a higher potential upside than MLCDs, I prefer MLCDs because they are less complex and offer an absolute principal guarantee, so this book will not explore market-linked notes.

Like traditional CDs, MLCDs also have a specific maturity date. But unlike traditional CDs, which pay a declared fixed interest rate each year, MLCDs pay interest that is tied to the performance of its underlying asset (market index, or basket of securities) over the full term of the MLCD. In other words, the investor won't know how much interest the MLCD will earn, if any, until it matures. If the underlying asset increases in value, the MLCD increases in value. If the underlying asset has a negative performance over the full term of the MLCD, the investor does not lose any money; they will get back 100% of their principal. Some of the available underlying asset categories are tied to major indexes, such as the S&P 500® or the Dow Jones Industrial Average (DJIA), while others are tied to a blend of indexes. Some underlying assets may use a combination of stock and bond indexes, and may attempt to limit market volatility by using "trend and equity volatility signals", driven by an algorithm, to determine the exposure to each of the indices, sometimes on a daily basis. "The market-linked CD can be tied to any index as long as the bank can purchase an option to adequately hedge the equity-linked interest payment."[6]

General MLCD Characteristics

- **Principal Protection and FDIC Insurance:** MLCDs are 100% principal protected when held to maturity. In addition, should the bank that issued the MLCD become insolvent, up to $250,000 of principal, per depositor, per depository institution, is guaranteed by FDIC Insurance. Earnings are not covered by FDIC insurance.

- **Term:** The term of the MLCD is generally 2-7 years.

- **Call Provision:** Some MLCDs have a call provision, which gives the bank the option of redeeming the investor's MLCD before the maturity date. Under that scenario, in addition to the principal, the investor would receive a call premium. A bank might call the MLCD if the underlying index has performed better than the stated call premium. It is solely the bank's discretion to exercise a call provision.

- **Participation Rate:** This rate is the percentage at which the total return corresponds to the performance of the underlying index. The participation rate may be less than or equal to 100% or greater than 100% and is set at issue. The MLCD's return is determined by multiplying the performance of the underlying index by the MLCD's participation rate. For example, if the participation rate of an MLCD is 150%, and the underlying asset has a positive return of 30% over the full term of the MLCD, the investor would receive 45% in interest credited to their MLCD (30% return x 150% participation rate = 45% interest).

- **Averaging Calculations:** To reduce the effects of market volatility, some MLCDs use an averaging method to calculate the return. With this method, the values of the underlying index are taken at various points along the term of the CD (normally near the end), and averaged. Averaging can work in favor of the investor or against the investor, depending on market conditions.

- **Caps:** Some MLCDs have a cap. A cap provides the maximum interest that the investor will receive at maturity. For example, if there is a 40% cap, the maximum interest paid at maturity is 40%. If the initial investment was $100,000, then the maximum the investor will receive at maturity is $140,000.

- **Minimum Interest Rate:** Some MLCDs guarantee a minimum interest rate regardless of the performance of the underlying asset. A minimum interest rate often reduces the potential upside of the MLCD.

- **Liquidity:** Because there is no secondary market for MLCDs, they generally should be held to maturity, or when called. Though a bank might make a market in their own offerings and buy back MLCDs before maturity, the investor is likely to receive less than their initial investment, depending on current interest rates and value of the option purchased by the bank. The value of the option is determined by market conditions, and the volatility of the underlying asset. As the MLCD nears its maturity, the value should get closer to face value. Again, if the MLCD is held to maturity, the investor will receive a minimum of 100% of their original investment. For example, if $100,000 were invested in the MLCD, then the minimum amount received at maturity will be $100,000.

- **Market Value:** The market value of the MLCD will fluctuate and might be less than the initial amount invested due to fees (including upfront costs), interest rates, underlying asset performance, market volatility, the length of the term, and how close it is to maturity.

- **Taxes:** Traditional CDs pay monthly interest, which is taxed each year as ordinary income. MLCDs, on the other hand, normally don't pay interest until maturity. So, you might expect that taxes are not due until maturity, when the interest is determined. Not so. MLCDs are taxed each year on "phantom income", which is non-existent income, equivalent to the interest paid by a traditional bank CD with a similar term. For example, if the MLCD has a 5-year term, there might be a 2% yearly phantom income attributed to the MLCD (assuming a 5-year traditional CD is yielding 2%.) Once the MLCD matures and any earned interest is determined, the investor will either owe additional taxes on the earnings, not owe any additional taxes, or receive a tax credit in the event the interest received is less than the amount taxed as phantom income. If held in an IRA, taxes on MLCDs are deferred, just like other assets held in an IRA.

MLCDs can be growth-oriented or income-oriented.

- **Growth-Oriented MLCDs** give the investor market exposure while maintaining principal protection. These investments may be appropriate for long-term investors seeking a potentially higher return than traditional CDs, money markets, savings accounts, and bonds. They may also be appropriate for an investor looking to reduce equity risk exposure in their portfolio.

- **Income-Structured MLCDs** pay interest coupons, like bonds, but the coupons aren't fixed. They are tied to changes in the underlying index and are not guaranteed. If an investor is looking for steady or guaranteed interest income, an income structured MLCD may not be appropriate.

Before investing, refer to the offering document of the MLCD for the terms, fees, and other important information.

Annuities

An annuity is a long-term investment issued by an insurance company that promises to pay income on a regular basis, for a specified period, or for the lifetime of the annuity owner. Like other forms of insurance, annuities can be simple or complex, with different types of annuities designed for different investors' needs. Annuities are often overlooked or criticized due to the general perception that they are expensive, illiquid, and complex. But if they are properly allocated and utilized, annuities can offer diversification, tax-deferred growth, income guarantees, principal protection, and a death benefit. Like all investments, annuities carry some risks, but when combined with an appropriate retirement planning strategy, they can provide insurance-like protection and steady income streams. Annuities are not appropriate for all investors, and the benefits, terms, and conditions should be carefully evaluated before deciding to purchase an annuity. Additionally, since annuity values (specifically fixed and index annuities) are backed by the insurance company, be sure to choose a financially sound company. You can review the insurance company's rating from four independent rating agencies, including:

- A.M. Best
- Standard & Poor's
- Moody's
- Fitch Ratings

There are two general categories of annuities: immediate and deferred.

Immediate Annuities

An immediate annuity, often referred to as a single premium immediate annuity (SPIA), is funded with a single lump-sum premium payment, and the income stream usually starts within 12 months after purchase. SPIAs offer a return in the form of interest, return of principal, and mortality credits (derived from annuitants who die early). This type of annuity (along with deferred income annuities, discussed later), provides a higher level of income than other forms of annuities. The main benefit of an SPIA is that it offers guaranteed fixed income, which can be payable over a specified period or for the life of the annuitant, reducing longevity risk. This is possible because a SPIA (and the annuitization of a deferred annuity, described later) is paid out of a pool of assets from a large group of annuitants, whose aggregate longevity is more predictable than an individual's anticipated longevity. On the downside, an investor gives up the rights to their principal and a death benefit in exchange for a guaranteed payment, so there's little flexibility. Another disadvantage is that the SPIA might not provide a rising income stream to keep pace with inflation. As discussed in Chapter 3, the income options of an SPIA include: single life option; joint and survivor option; or a period certain option. The election of an installment refund for single life and joint and survivor options results in continued payments to beneficiaries for a specified period, even after the death of the annuitant (and spouse, if a joint and survivor option was chosen). The election of a cash refund results in a lump sum payment of the unpaid amount to the beneficiaries. These extra guarantees will result in an initial lower income payment.

As discussed in Chapter 5, SPIAs can be funded with qualified (pre-tax) or non-qualified (after-tax) money. If funded with qualified money, all income is taxable as ordinary income. If funded with non-qualified money, part of the income will be treated as a tax-free return of principal, while a portion will be treated as taxable interest, subject to ordinary income taxes. The calculation is based on an "exclusion ratio". Once the principal has been fully paid out, all future income is taxable.

Deferred Annuities

A deferred annuity can be funded with a single lump-sum premium payment, or with an initial premium payment followed by additional premium payments over time. Deferred annuities have an accumulation period and a payout (or distribution) period, during which the annuity owner receives income from the annuity. The annuity can earn a fixed rate of interest, an interest rate based on the growth of an external index or can increase in value by the growth of the subaccounts. Distributions are usually deferred until some point in the future, such as retirement. Distributions from a deferred annuity can be a lump sum payment, a series of payments, or through annuitization (the process of converting an annuity into a series of periodic income payments, which pays principal, interest, and mortality credits over a specified period, or for the annuitant's life). Similar to a SPIA, annuitization options include a single life option, a joint and survivor option, or a period certain option. The election of an installment refund for single life and joint and survivor options results in continued payments to beneficiaries for a specified period, even after the death of the annuity owner (and spouse, if a joint and survivor option was chosen). The election of a cash refund results in a lump sum payment of the unpaid amount to the beneficiaries. As with SPIAs, these extra guarantees will result in an initial lower income payment.

Although annuitization is one of the distribution choices, most annuity contracts are never annuitized, because the rights to the annuity's principal are permanently granted to the insurance company. Because of this disadvantage, most annuity owners take withdrawals from their annuities without annuitizing their contracts. Due to the possibility of depleting the annuity value and outliving those withdrawals, some annuities offer an optional guaranteed withdrawal benefit rider or income rider for an additional fee. This rider guarantees income payments for an individual and can also guarantee income payments for a surviving spouse. Some annuities also offer an enhanced death benefit for an additional fee. These optional riders will be discussed later in this chapter.

Deferred annuities are normally subject to a surrender charge for early withdrawal, typically a declining charge that lasts from 5-10 years or longer. During the surrender charge period, most annuities allow penalty-free withdrawals, normally 10% of the annuity value. Annuities could also be subject to a market value adjustment (MVA), which reduces the value of the withdrawal should interest rates go up, and which increases the value of the withdrawal should interest rates go down. The purpose of the MVA is to discourage the annuity owner from taking large withdrawals to reinvest elsewhere, should interest rates increase. The MVA usually disappears when there are no longer any surrender charges. Annuities are meant to be long-term investments often used to provide supplemental retirement income.

Deferred annuities can be funded with qualified (pre-tax) or non-qualified (after-tax) money. However funded, earnings on deferred annuities are tax-deferred. Please note that purchasing an annuity within an IRA or retirement plan - which are already tax-deferred - provides no additional tax benefits. Some additional tax considerations include:

- If the annuity is funded with qualified money, all distributions are taxable as ordinary income, regardless of the method chosen. If withdrawals are taken prior to age 59½, the entire amount of the withdrawal could be subject to a 10% IRS penalty. The death benefit is fully taxable to your heirs.

- If the annuity is funded with non-qualified money, when withdrawals (other than annuitization) are taken, the earnings portion, which is taxable as ordinary income, comes out first (LIFO - Last In, First Out), followed by principal. If the annuity is annuitized, part of the income is treated as a tax-free return of principal, while a portion is treated as earnings and subject to ordinary income taxes. The calculation is based on an exclusion ratio. Once the principal has been fully paid out, all future income is taxable. This is similar to the taxation of an immediate annuity. If withdrawals are taken prior to age 59½, the earnings portion could be subject to a 10% IRS penalty. The earnings portion of the death benefit is taxable to your heirs.

There are three types of deferred annuities: fixed, indexed and variable.

Fixed Annuities

Fixed annuities (FAs) offer guarantee of principal by the insurance company and pay a fixed interest rate for a period of either one year or multiple years. After the initial guarantee, the FA will set another fixed interest rate for the next rate period. It could be higher or lower than the previous rate, depending on interest rates paid by bonds at the time of renewal. (Insurance companies invest the annuity owner's premium payments in bonds.) FAs usually offer a minimum guaranteed interest rate. Some FAs offer a premium bonus, which is a lump sum added to the annuity by the insurance company at the time of purchase or when money is added by the owner. Other FAs offer an interest bonus, which is a higher interest rate to attract new buyers. While these "bonuses" might sound attractive, they usually come at a price. Interest bonuses could be lost if money is withdrawn before a set period of time. In addition, the renewal rates could be lower than that of an annuity without a bonus. FAs are the most conservative type of deferred annuities.

Deferred Income Annuities

A newer type of fixed annuity is called a deferred income annuity (DIA). A DIA is similar in structure to an SPIA, but it is designed as longevity insurance, as it ensures the payout of additional lifetime income if a person lives beyond a certain age. While life insurance pays a death benefit, protecting against the risk of dying too soon, a DIA pays an income stream starting at a selected payout date, protecting against the risk of living too long. The DIA works like an SPIA - the income payments combine interest, return of principal, and mortality credits. The main difference is that DIAs start paying income as early as 13 months after purchase, or as far out as 30-40 years (depending on your age and insurance company), while SPIAs normally start paying income within 12 months after purchase. A DIA can be purchased as a qualified annuity (pre-tax), or a non-qualified annuity (after-tax). Income taxation is the same as immediate annuities. The main advantage of a DIA is that it pays a guaranteed lifetime income starting at a specified date in the future, so it protects against longevity risk. The disadvantages are similar to SPIAs: no right to principal, might not keep up with inflation, etc. Another consideration is, what happens if you die before you start receiving payments, or only after a few years, when the total of the payments received is less than what you contributed into the annuity? To deal with this risk, most insurance companies offer a return of premium option, which guarantees that your beneficiaries will receive the premiums paid, minus any withdrawals.

Fixed Indexed Annuities

Fixed Indexed Annuities (FIAs) are a type of fixed annuity that earns interest based on the changes of a market index, such as the S&P 500®, Nasdaq 100, Russell 2000, or another index. FIAs are not directly invested in the "underlying" market index, so dividends are not paid. But these types of annuities will never suffer market losses and credited interest is never less than zero, even if the index value declines. Most FIAs include a fixed rate account with competitive interest rates. These annuities were designed for the investor looking to earn higher interest rates (than other fixed annuities) by being linked to market indexes without any downside risk. For example, an FIA is purchased on July 1 in year 1, and all the assets are initially allocated to an S&P 500® Index fund using an annual point-to-point calculation (beginning index value to ending index value). Let's assume that on July 1 of the first year, the S&P 500® Index is at 3000, and on July 1 of the following year, the S&P 500® Index is at 3300. The one-year return would be calculated by subtracting the beginning value from the ending value, and then dividing that figure by the beginning value: 3300 - 3000 = 300; 300 / 3000 = 10%.

FIAs typically include controls imposed by the issuing insurance company, limiting the maximum interest rate credited. These include:

- A cap, which limits the index increase to determine the interest credited

- A spread, which is deducted from the index increase to determine the interest credited
- A participation rate, which is a percentage of the index increase to determine the interest credited

Some insurance companies offer all three options, while others limit the options to one or two choices. In the previous example, with the S&P 500® return of 10%, if the annuity had a cap rate of 6%, the interest credited would be 6%. If the spread was 3%, then the interest credited would be 7% (10% - 3% = 7%). Lastly, if the participation rate was 50%, the interest credited would be 5% (10% x 50% = 5%). No single crediting method consistently provides the highest interest under all market conditions. Participation rates could have a higher potential upside than caps or spreads in years when index returns are higher. Some FIAs include indexes that may use a combination of stock and bond indexes, and may attempt to limit market volatility by using "trend and equity volatility signals", driven by an algorithm, to determine the exposure to each of the indices, sometimes on a daily basis. These indexes may offer a higher cap or participation rate than a more standard index, such as the S&P 500®. Allocations to the market indexes are chosen when the annuity is purchased and can usually be reallocated on the contract anniversary. It bears repeating that because FIAs are not invested directly in the market or the index, interest credited does not include any dividends.

A major benefit of FIAs is guarantee of principal. So, for instance, in the previous example, if the S&P 500® had dropped from 3000-2700, the index itself would have lost 10%. But because FIAs have no market risk, the interest credited would be 0% for that year, and the annuity would not decline in value. The tradeoff for the protection from market downturns is the limited growth potential.

Insurance companies use different formulas to calculate how the interest is determined, including:

- **Annual Point-to-Point:** Measured by the change in the index over a one-year period.

- **Multi-Year Point-to-Point:** Measured by the change in the index over a multi-year period.

- **Monthly or Daily Averaging:** Monthly averaging is measured by taking the average value of the index on a specific day each month; daily averaging is measured by taking the average index value each day that the market is open. For each of these averaging methods, the average value is compared with the starting index value (i.e., S&P 500®) to determine the interest credited.

- **Monthly Point-to-Point:** Measured by the change in the index for each month over a one-year period. Each monthly change is limited to the index cap rate for positive changes, but there is no limit for negative changes. At the end of the one-year period, all monthly changes (both positive and negative) are added. If the ending result is positive, the interest is added to the annuity. If the ending result is zero or negative, no interest is added.

Automatic Annual Reset

Annual reset is a common feature and a major benefit of FIAs. With this feature, the annuity's index values are automatically reset at the end of the contract year, and the year's ending index value becomes the next year's starting value. In addition, the interest earned during the contract year is "locked in" as part of the annuity's value and cannot be lost in the future. Each year, as the annuity increases in value, the ending (higher) value - which includes any credited interest - is automatically "reset" as the next year's starting value. So, you can never lose previous year's earned interest. With an annual reset, the worst-case scenario is the annuity retains its value in any year that the index is negative. For example, let's assume an initial investment of $100,000 in an annual point-to-point index with a cap of 5%. If the index is up 10%, at the end of the first contract anniversary, the value of the FIA would be $105,000, minus any fees (if any). Even if the index loses 10% in the following year, the value of the FIA would remain at $105,000, minus any fees (if any). With other types of investments, you could enjoy large gains one year, only to lose them the next year. This is an important distinction from investing directly in the stock market. From 2003-2007, the S&P 500® had five straight years of positive returns, only to give back a large portion of those gains in 2008, when it lost 37%. With an FIA, you most likely would have had the same five straight years of positive returns (subject to caps, spreads, or participation rates, discussed earlier), but in 2008, instead of losing 37%, your return would have been 0%, a significant downside protection from market losses. Contrarily, in periods of higher stock market returns, such as from 2009-2019, FIAs could have significantly underperformed the stock market, due to their upside limitations. But for those investors who cannot afford to lose money, or who do not want to subject their money to the ups and downs of the stock market, these types of annuities can be very appealing.

Variable Annuities

Variable Annuities (VAs) are a type of annuity that earns investment returns based on the performance of its investment accounts, known as "subaccounts," which can be invested in stock, bond, or money market funds. The value of the subaccounts changes daily, based on changes in the markets, so these annuities do involve investment risk and can lose money. Subaccounts are like mutual funds and can be passively or actively managed. Some VAs offer a guaranteed fixed interest subaccount. Unlike an FA or FIA, where the investment risk is carried by the insurance company, with a VA, the investment risk falls on the annuity owner.

VAs are often criticized for having high fees. They typically have a mortality and expense annual charge of 1-1.5%, the average being 1.25%. This fee is imposed to offset the cost to the insurer of any income guarantees that are included in the annuity contract. The insurer's costs and risks typically involve the owner's right to annuitize the contract (providing payments of principal and interest over an annuitant's lifetime), the guaranteed death benefit (which could be higher than the contract value or greater than the premiums paid into the contract), and a guarantee that the contract expenses won't increase. The mortality and expense fee is a percentage of the annuity's value, but is typically not charged on the guaranteed interest subaccount. VAs also incur annual management fees for each subaccount, typically ranging from .5-2.0%, the average being 1%.

Some of the advantages of a variable annuity include: tax deferral (unless it is funded with qualified, pre-tax money, as it would already have the tax deferral benefit), the ability to move money from one subaccount to another without any tax consequences, no upside limits, and the ability to annuitize the contract for a guaranteed lifetime income.

Index Variable Annuities

Newer versions of VAs offered by a number of insurance companies, called Index Variable Annuities (IVAs), offer the ability to participate in market gains with some level of protection against market losses. Annuity owners can choose the index or indexes to allocate to, such as the S&P 500® Index, Nasdaq 100 Index, Russell 2000 Index, MSCI EAFE Index, or other indexes. Just like FIAs, IVAs are not directly invested in the "underlying" market index, so dividends are not paid. IVAs allow the annuity owner to choose a crediting method that includes a cap rate, along with a corresponding "buffer" rate or a "floor" rate that limits negative index returns. A "buffer" absorbs a fixed percentage of losses in the index. For example, if the buffer is 10%, the annuity owner is not subject to the first 10% of losses in the index, only to any losses beyond 10%. So, if the index falls 25%, the losses in the IVA would be limited to 15% (25% loss - 10% buffer = 15%). A "floor," on the other hand, limits negative index returns up to a certain percentage. For example, if the floor is 10%, the annuity owner is subject to the first 10% of losses in the index, but is not subject to any losses beyond that. So, if the index falls 25%, the losses in the IVA would be limited to 10%.

IVAs typically have higher cap rates than FIAs, so they do have a higher upside potential than FIAs, but they usually don't offer the same downside protection. IVAs typically carry fees, but they are often lower than those of traditional VAs since the index itself does not carry a fee. If you are looking for some downside protection, IVAs may be more appealing than traditional VAs since they offer some downside protection and lower fees. But the tradeoff will be lower upside potential than VAs, which don't cap earnings. Some IVAs allow the annuity owner to lock in gains before the contract anniversary.

When evaluating IVAs and FIAs, something to consider is that most IVAs do not lock in annual compounded gains, as FIAs do. While the IVA offers some downside protection, this protection resets on the contract anniversary. For example, assuming a $100,000 initial investment in an IVA with a 10% floor and a cap rate of 10%, if, in the first year, the S&P 500® index is up 10%, the value of the IVA would increase to $110,000 before fees. If the index were to drop 10% in the second year, the value of the IVA would decrease to $99,000 before fees, wiping out all the gains from the previous year. Now let's look at the same investment in an FIA. Again, assuming a $100,000 initial investment in an FIA with a 5% cap, if, in the first year, the S&P 500® index is up 10%, the value of the FIA would increase to $105,000 before fees. If the index were to drop 10% in the second year, the value of the FIA would remain at $105,000 before fees, and all the gains from the previous year are retained. This can make an FIA more appealing than an IVA, since gains are locked in every year and can never be subject to any market losses.

Optional Guaranteed Withdrawal Benefit Rider/Income Rider

With people living longer, and U.S. companies shifting away from defined benefit pension plans, retirees are left with fewer sources of guaranteed lifetime income, but a greater need for them, as they face longevity risk – the risk that they will outlive their money. While an SPIA, DIA, or the annuitization of a deferred annuity can fill this gap, these options normally don't offer the flexibility of stopping and restarting payments. Nor do they normally offer a rising income to keep pace with inflation. As an alternative, some FAs, FIAs, IVAs, and VAs offer an optional guaranteed withdrawal benefit rider or a guaranteed income rider for an additional fee. These riders guarantee income payments for life. If you are married, a joint income rider would guarantee income payments for as long as either you or your spouse live. With a rider, if you die (or if both you and your spouse die with a joint income rider) before or while receiving income payments, your survivors will receive the death benefit (provided it is greater than $0). If the income payments reduce the annuity's cash value to $0, you (and your spouse, if you have a joint income rider) will continue to receive income payments for life. If the annuity owner takes additional lump sum withdrawals or a larger income payment than the rider allows, it could impact the guarantees of the rider. Some riders provide the potential for income increases over time, to help keep pace with inflation.

Optional Death Benefit Rider

Some annuities offer several choices of death benefit options. The traditional or basic death benefit typically pays the greater of the contract value or total premium purchase payments, adjusted by any withdrawals on the death of the annuitant. An optional death benefit rider, offered for an additional fee, may lock in the death benefit value on each contract anniversary. These riders vary by insurance company and by annuity. If the primary goal of the annuity is to leave a legacy, an optional death benefit rider may be worth adding.

Considerations of an Annuity

While a fixed annuity (FA) and fixed index annuity (FIA) may be most appealing to a conservative investor, a variable annuity (VA) may be most appealing to a more aggressive investor, and an index variable annuity (IVA) may be appealing to a moderate investor. If the annuity is purchased for the primary purpose of providing an income stream in retirement, consider a SPIA or a DIA, and consider adding an optional guaranteed withdrawal benefit rider/income rider to a deferred annuity. If the intention is to leave the annuity as a legacy, consider adding an optional death benefit rider.

Annuities offer many benefits, but can be complex. Make sure you fully understand what you are buying before you commit to it; this includes the guarantees and risks of the annuity. If you are working with a financial advisor or insurance broker, they should have a good understanding of your personal and financial position before recommending an annuity, and should be able to explain the annuity in detail, including the fees, limitations, and how the riders work. Since all product guarantees depend on the insurance company's financial strength and claims-paying ability, stick with highly rated insurance companies licensed to do business in your state.

Alternative Strategy Mutual Funds, ETFs, and Separately Managed Accounts

For investors looking to reduce risk in their investment portfolios, there are many alternative strategy mutual funds, exchange traded funds (ETFs), and separately managed accounts (SMAs) to consider. Unlike typical equity funds that remain fully invested in stock or bonds during both up and down markets, these funds use various strategies to become defensive in market downturns, with the goal of preserving capital and limiting losses. Some examples of these strategies include:

- Funds that reduce equity exposure, by shifting from stocks to bonds or cash during periods of market stress.

- Funds that utilize managed futures (long and short, depending on market conditions). Managed futures have historically performed well in periods of market stress.

- Funds that use other sophisticated strategies to reduce market risk.

While these strategies can potentially lower the risk in a portfolio, they offer no guarantees against loss of principal, and no assurances that they will achieve their investment objective. In addition, there may be periods of time when they underperform their benchmarks. Still, they may be appropriate for some investors, especially if they give the investor the confidence to remain invested in times of market volatility.

Summary

As a recap, for the conservative investor, or the investor seeking to reduce market risk and preserve capital, some suitable investments to consider include: market-linked CDs (MLCDs), fixed annuities (FAs), fixed index annuities (FIAs), index variable annuities (IVAs), and alternative strategy mutual funds/exchange traded funds (ETFs)/separately managed accounts (SMAs). For the retiree seeking consistent, guaranteed income, single premium immediate annuities (SPIAs), deferred income annuities (DIAs), or deferred annuities with an optional guaranteed withdrawal benefit rider or income rider may be suitable investments to consider. Investors who employ strategies for protecting principal, reducing downside risk, and providing guaranteed lifetime income can be prepared for any scenario before or during retirement. Of course, it is best to consider your individual goals, financial circumstances, risk tolerance, and tax situation when making investment decisions.

PART II SUMMARY

Part II starts off with a discussion on developing a retirement income plan. It continues with a discussion of the various risks faced in retirement including:

- Healthcare spending risk
- Long-term care risk
- The death or divorce of a spouse/partner
- Not having a proper estate plan
- Taxes in retirement
- Bad advice, scams, fraud, and identity theft
- Longevity risk
- Withdrawal risk
- Sequence of return risk
- Investment risk
- Investment behavior

Various suggestions are discussed to mitigate these risks, including a final chapter on financial risk management strategies. These strategies can be implemented to help reduce specific retirement risks including longevity risk, withdrawal risk, sequence of return risk, investment risk, and investment behavior. As with Part I, these suggestions don't need to be applied all at once. The key is to choose the items that are most important to you and to start there.

Since the intention of this book is to provide investment education, no specific product recommendations are discussed. Please speak to your financial advisor to learn more about the strategies discussed in this book or contact me through my website, https://www.luongowealthmanagement.com/, with any questions.

REFERENCES

Part I

Introduction

1. Ruth Sackman, *Rethinking Cancer: Non-Traditional Approaches to the Theories, Treatments and Prevention of Cancer* (Garden City Park: Square One Publishers, 2003), 5.

Chapter 1

1. "Health, United States, 2018 - Data Finder." Centers for Disease Control and Prevention, 30 Oct. 2019, https://www.cdc.gov/nchs/hus/contents2018.htm?search=Life_expectancy.
2. Police, Sara. *"How Much Have Obesity Rates Risen Since 1950?"* LIVESTRONG.COM, Leaf Group, https://www.livestrong.com/article/384722-how-much-have-obesity-rates-risen-since-1950/.
3. Murray, Christopher J.L., et al., "The Vast Majority of American Adults Are Overweight or Obese, and Weight Is a Growing Problem Among US Children." *Institute for Health Metrics and Evaluation,* 27 Nov. 2018, http://www.healthdata.org/news-release/vast-majority-american-adults-are-overweight-or-obese-and-weight-growing-problem-among.
4. Sackman, *Rethinking Cancer,* 17.

Chapter 2

1. "Genetically Modified Organism." *Wikipedia,* Wikimedia Foundation, 18 Nov. 2019, https://en.wikipedia.org/wiki/Genetically_modified_organism.
2. Sackman, *Rethinking Cancer,* 17.
3. Peter D'Adamo and Catherine Whitney, *Eat Right 4 Your Type: The Original Individualized Blood Type Diet Solution,* (New York: Arrow Books, 2016), 5.
4. Deville, Lauren. "Hydrochloric Acid and Your Blood Type: Naturopathic Doctor - Tucson, AZ", 1 Feb. 2019, https://www.drlaurendeville.com/articles/hydrochloric-acid-and-your-blood-type/.

5. Ramsey, Glenn E., "What Does Your Blood Type Mean for Your Health?," *Northwestern Medicine*, https://www.nm.org/healthbeat/healthy-tips/what-does-your-blood-type-mean-for-your-health.
6. Ramsey, *What Does Your Blood Type Mean*.

Chapter 3

1. "Indoor Air Quality." *EPA*, Environmental Protection Agency, 16 July 2018, https://www.epa.gov/report-environment/indoor-air-quality.
2. Vartan, Starre. "Easy Ways to Clear Your Indoor Air." *Chicagotribune.com*, 23 May 2019, https://www.chicagotribune.com/real-estate/ct-xpm-2012-01-20-sc-home-0116-indoor-air-20120120-story.html.
3. Van Den Wymelenberg, PhD, Kevin. "Sunlight Reduces Harmful Bacteria Inside Your House." *Bottom Line Personal*, 3 Mar. 2019.
4. Simon, Stacy. "How to Test Your Home for Radon." *American Cancer Society*, 29 Oct. 2019, https://www.cancer.org/latest-news/radon-gas-and-lung-cancer.html.

Chapter 4

1. Brownstein MD, David. "How to Stop Environmental Toxins From Poisoning You", *Natural Way to Health*, Mar. 2012, Vol. 5, Issue 3, 1.
2. Vartan, Starre. "Easy Ways to Clear Your Indoor Air." *Chicagotribune.com*, 23 May 2019, https://www.chicagotribune.com/real-estate/ct-xpm-2012-01-20-sc-home-0116-indoor-air-20120120-story.html.
3. Pope, Sarah MGA. "Roundup: Quick Death for Weeds, Slow Death for You - Healthy Home." *The Healthy Home Economist*, 20 May 2019, https://www.thehealthyhomeeconomist.com/roundup-quick-death-for-weeds-slow-and-painful-death-for-you.
4. Gelula, Melisse. "Fragrance Ingredients: What You Need to Know." *Well+Good*, 27 June 2018, https://www.wellandgood.com/ingredient-intelligence-what-you-need-to-know-about-fragrance-in-skin-care/.
5. Rodale, Maria. "Five 'Must-Knows' on the Dangers of Synthetic Fragrance." *HuffPost*, 7 Dec. 2017, https://www.huffpost.com/entry/five-mustknows-on-the-dan_b_4737654?guccounter=1.
6. Milman, Oliver. "US cosmetics are full of chemicals banned by Europe – why?" *The Guardian*, 22 May 2019, https://www.theguardian.com/us-news/2019/may/22/chemicals-in-cosmetics-us-restricted-eu.
7. "Top Ten Reasons to Oppose Water Fluoridation." *IAOMT*, The International Academy of Oral Medicine & Toxicology, 3 Dec. 2018, https://

iaomt.org/top-ten-reasons-oppose-water-fluoridation/.
8. Brownstein, Stop Environmental Toxins, 5.
9. Brownstein MD, David, "Aluminum: The Poison All Around Us", *Natural Way to Health,* May 2016, Vol. 9, Issue 5, 2-3
10. Brownstein, Stop Environmental Toxins, 2.
11. Liz, "Is Your Mattress Toxic? Symptoms and Solutions", *Savvy Rest,* https://savvyrest.com/blog/your-mattress-toxic-symptoms-solutions#:~:text=Chemical%20Off%2DGassing,-One%20of%20the&text=Flame%20retardants%2C%20formaldehyde%2C%20and%20benzene,-toxins%20for%20hours%20every%20night.

Chapter 5

1. Joseph Mercola, *Effortless Healing: 9 Simple Ways to Sidestep Illness, Shed Excess Weight, and Help Your Body Fix Itself,* (New York: Harmony Crown, 2015), 134.
2. Ibid., 129-136.
3. "Vitamin D Deficiency: 6 Causes, Common Symptoms & Health Risks." *WebMD,* 16 May 2018, https://www.webmd.com/diet/guide/vitamin-d-deficiency#1.
4. Brownstein MD, David "The Powerful Nutrient That's Right in Your Backyard", *Natural Way to Health,* October 2011, Vol. 4, Issue 10, 3, 5.
5. Vitamin D Deficiency.

Chapter 6

1. Sackman, *Rethinking Cancer,* 64.
2. Ann Boroch, *Healing Multiple Sclerosis: Diet, Detox & Nutritional Makeover for Total Recovery,* (Los Angeles: Quintessential Healing Publishing, 2014), 97.
3. Ibid., 163-169.
4. Mercola, *Effortless Healing,* 198, 200.
5. Boroch, *Healing Multiple Sclerosis,* 164-165.
6. Camo, Bonnie, *Natural Medicine,* 2018, 171.
7. Petersen, Julie. "How Technology Makes You Stressed." *Goalcast,* 19 Sept. 2019, https://www.goalcast.com/2017/02/13/technology-makes-stressed/.

Chapter 7

1. "What Is Sleep?" *Popular Science - The Science of Sleep*, 2019, 9.
2. Mercola, *Effortless Healing*, 181-182.
3. "Common Sleep Disorders." *Popular Science - The Science of Sleep*, 2019, 36.
4. Ibid., 36-37.
5. Mercola, *Effortless Healing*, 175-192.
6. "Tips and Hacks to Get Better Z's." *Popular Science - The Science of Sleep*, 2019, 78-79.

Chapter 8

1. Mercola, *Effortless Healing*, 108.
2. Phillips, Stuart M. "Surefire Ways to Prevent Muscle Loss." *Bottom Line Personal*, 1 Mar. 2019.
3. Mercola, *Effortless Healing*, 118.
4. Ibid., 120.
5. D'Adamo and Whitney, *Eat Right 4 Your Type*, 125-126.
6. Ibid., 165-166.
7. Ibid., 200-201.
8. Ibid., 236-237.
9. Sackman, *Rethinking Cancer*, 65.

Chapter 9

1. Brownstein MD, David "A Simple Way To Radically Improve Your Health", *Natural Way to Health,* June 2009, Vol. 2, Issue 6, 2.
2. Mercola, *Effortless Healing*, 41.
3. Readfearn, Graham. "WHO Launches Health Review after Microplastics Found in 90% of Bottled Water." *The Guardian*, Guardian News and Media, 15 Mar. 2018, https://www.theguardian.com/environment/2018/mar/15/microplastics-found-in-more-than-90-of-bottled-water-study-says.
4. Boyles, Salynn. "Bottled Water: FAQ on Safety and Purity." *WebMD*, 7 Nov. 2008, https://www.webmd.com/food-recipes/news/20081107/bottled-water-faq-on-safety-and-purity#1.
5. Ibid.
6. "The Environmental Impacts of Plastic Water Bottles." *Go Green*, 14 Nov. 2017, http://www.gogreen.org/blog/impacts-of-plastic-water-bottles.

Chapter 10

1. Brownstein MD, David "Probiotics: Secret Ingredient for Better Health", *Natural Way to Health,* Nov. 2014, Vol. 7, Issue 11, 3.
2. "The Difference Between Good Bacteria and Bad Bacteria", *Humm Kombucha,* 2019, https://hummkombucha.com/the-difference-between-good-bacteria-and-bad-bacteria/#:~:text=One%20of%20 the%20most%20well,bacteria%20and%2015%25%20bad%20bacteria.
3. Brownstein MD, David "Probiotics: Secret Ingredient for Better Health", *Natural Way to Health,* November 2014, Vol. 7, Issue 11, 2.
4. Mercola, Effortless Healing, 160-163.
5. Ibid., 169.
6. Brownstein MD, David "Fighting Viral Infections", *Natural Way to Health,* April 2020, Vol. 13, Issue 4, 4.

Chapter 11

1. Camo, Bonnie, MD. "The Truth about Fat and Carbs." *Natural Medicine,* 2018, 23.
2. West, Sarah. "Our Soils Are in Trouble and Organic Farming Can Help." *Nature's Path,* 22 June 2017, https://www.naturespath.com/en-us/blog/our-soils-are-in-trouble-and-organic-farming-can-help/.
3. "What Is a GMO?" *NON GMO Project,* https://www.nongmoproject.org/gmo-facts/what-is-gmo/.
4. Bayer AG. "Biotechnology and GMOs." *Bayer,* 23 Apr. 2019, https://www.bayer.com/en/crop-science-innovations-biotech-gmos.aspx.
5. "GMO Science." *NON GMO Project,* https://www.nongmoproject.org/gmo-facts/science/.
6. Bellon, Tina. "California Jury Hits Bayer With $2 Billion Award in Roundup Cancer Trial", 19 May, 2019, https://www.reuters.com/article/us-bayer-glyphosate-lawsuit/california-jury-hits-bayer-with-2-billion-award-in-roundup-cancer-trial-idUSKCN1SJ29F.
7. Mercola, *Effortless Healing,* 89.
8. Schaefer, Anna and Yasin, Kareem, "Experts Agree: Sugar Might Be as Addictive as Cocaine", https://www.healthline.com/health/food-nutrition/experts-is-sugar-addictive-drug.
9. Mercola, Effortless Healing, 89.
10. "56 Different Names for Sugars Hiding on Food Labels." *Cityline,* 26 July 2019, https://www.cityline.tv/2017/06/14/56-names-sugars-havent-heard/.

11. Brownstein MD, David "5 Common Foods That Damage Your Health", *Natural Way to Health,* November 2014, Vol. 7, Issue 11, p. 2.
12. Amit. "Is Whole Wheat Bread Really Better Than White Bread?" *The Bread Guide,* 15 Sept. 2019, https://thebreadguide.com/whole-wheat-or-white-bread/.
13. David Perlmutter, MD, *Grain Brain* (New York: Little, Brown and Company, 2013), 8.
14. Brownstein MD, David "Cereals Contaminated with Weed Killer", *Natural Way to Health,* March 2019, Vol. 12, Issue 3, 6.
15. Brownstein MD, David "Soft Drinks Are Sweetly Destroying Your Body", *Natural Way to Health,* April 2011, Vol. 4, Issue 4, 3.
16. Ibid., 7. p. 7.
17. David Brownstein, MD, and Sheryl Shenefelt, CN, *The Guide to Healthy Eating* (Healthy Living, 2010), 53.
18. Brownstein MD, David. "Low-Fat Foods Are Making You Fat", *Natural Way to Health,* August 2014, Vol. 7, Issue 8, 3.
19. Anthony Gustin and Emily Ziedman. "What's The Ideal Omega 3-6-9 Ratio?" *Perfect Keto,* 13 Sept. 2019, https://perfectketo.com/omega-3-6-9-ratio/.
20. Hari, Vani. "Processed To Death - Get These Cooking Oils Out of Your Pantry STAT!" *Food Babe,* 18 Sept. 2018, https://foodbabe.com/cooking-oils/.
21. Brownstein MD, David "Exposing the Dairy Myth: The Truth About Milk and Your Health", *Natural Way to Health,* November 2009, Vol. 2, Issue 11, 7.
22. Brownstein MD, David "Low-Fat Foods Are Making You Fat", *Natural Way to Health,* August 2014, Vol. 7, Issue 8, 5.
23. Brownstein MD, David "The American Paradox: How We Eat Ourselves Sick", *Natural Way to Health,* August 2010, Vol. 3, Issue 8, 3, 5.
24. "About GE Foods." *Center for Food Safety,* https://www.centerforfoodsafety.org/issues/311/ge-foods/about-ge-foods.
25. Brownstein and Sheneflet, *Healthy Eating,* 75.
26. Brownstein MD, David "Dangers and Misconceptions About Soy and Your Health", *Natural Way to Health,* December 2008, Vol. 1, Issue 8, 3.
27. Brownstein MD, David "Soy Good For You? Not So Fast", *Natural Way to Health,* November 2011, Vol. 4, Issue 11, p. 2.
28. Ibid., 3.
29. Brownstein MD, David "7 Simple Ways to Achieve Your Best Health", *Natural Way to Health,* January 2013, Vol. 6, Issue 1, 3.
30. Brownstein MD, David "Don't Believe the 'No-Salt' Myth", *Natural Way to*

Health, September 2011, Vol. 4, Issue 9, 3.
31. Brownstein and Shenefelt, *Healthy Eating,* 101.
32. "EWG's 2019 Shopper's Guide to Pesticides in Produce™." *EWG's 2019 Shopper's Guide to Pesticides in Produce | Summary,* 20 Mar. 2019, https://www.ewg.org/foodnews/summary.php.
33. Brownstein, "7 Simple Ways", 3.
34. Ibid., 3.
35. D'Adamo and Whitney, *Eat Right 4 Your Type,* 39-40.
36. Ibid., 50.
37. Ibid., 77.
38. https://www.papajohns.com/company/papa-johns-ingredients.html.
39. Marinaccio, Tina. "Bottom Line Personal." 15 Jan. 2019.
40. Mercola, *Effortless Healing,* 95.
41. Marinaccio, Tina. "Bottom Line Personal." 15 Jan. 2019.
42. Mercola, *Effortless Healing,* 96-98.

Chapter 12

1. Brownstein MD, David "A Holistic Doctor Can Change Your Life", *Natural Way to Health,* June 2012, Vol. 5, Issue 6, 1.
2. Ibid.
3. Brownstein MD, David "Too Much Medicine Will Kill You", *Natural Way to Health,* June 2019, Vol. 12, Issue 6, 1.
4. Cornejo, Corinna. "Patient Engagement and the Promise of Better Outcomes." *WEGOHEALTH,* https://www.wegohealth.com/2018/01/08/patient-engagement/.
5. Brownstein MD, David "Beware: Vitamin B6 Is a Double-Edged Sword", *Natural Way to Health,* June 2020, Vol. 13, Issue 6, 1.
6. Ibid., 3.
7. Perlmutter, *Grain Brain,* 41-42.
8. Brownstein MD, David "Achieve Optimal Health Through Holistic Dental Care", *Natural Way to Health,* September 2009, Vol. 2, Issue 9, 1.
9. Ibid., 2.
10. Ibid., 3.
11. Ibid., 3.
12. Brownstein MD, David "Root Canal: Danger to Your Whole Body", *Natural Way to Health,* April 2016, Vol. 9, Issue 4, 3.

Chapter 13

1. "Lifetime Risk of Developing or Dying From Cancer." *American Cancer Society,* https://www.cancer.org/cancer/cancer-basics/lifetime-probability-of-developing-or-dying-from-cancer.html.
2. Brownstein MD, David "7 Simple Steps to Prevent Cancer", *Natural Way to Health,* October 2012, Special Issue, 1.
3. "Cancer Facts & Figures 2018", https://www.cancer.org/content/dam/cancer-org/research/cancer-facts-and-statistics/annual-cancer-facts-and-figures/2018/cancer-facts-and-figures-2018.pdf.
4. Nall, Rachel. "Cancer: Overview, Causes, Treatments, and Types." *Medical News Today,* MediLexicon International, 12 Nov. 2018, https://www.medicalnewstoday.com/articles/323648.
5. Sackman, Rethinking Cancer, 3.
6. Brownstein MD, David, "Integrative Medicine Offers Cutting-Edge Cancer Treatments", *Natural Way to Health,* January 2019, Vol. 12, Issue 1, 7.
7. "Cancer Costs Projected to Reach at Least $158 Billion in 2020." *National Institutes of Health,* U.S. Department of Health and Human Services, 12 Jan. 2011, https://www.nih.gov/news-events/news-releases/cancer-costs-projected-reach-least-158-billion-2020#:~:text=Based%20on%20growth%20and%20aging,National%20Institutes%20of%20Health%20analysis..
8. Brownstein MD, David "New Holistic Health Tools to Find and Defeat Cancer", *Natural Way to Health,* January 2010, Vol. 3, Issue 1, 2.
9. Ibid., 2-3.
10. Sackman, Rethinking Cancer, 23-24.
11. Ibid., 127-128.

Chapter 16

1. Sherman, Erik. "U.S. Health Care Costs Skyrocketed to $3.65 Trillion in 2018." *Fortune,* 21 Feb. 2019, https://fortune.com/2019/02/21/us-health-care-costs-2/.
2. Radu, Sintia. "Countries With the Most Well-Developed Public Health Care Systems." *U.S. News & World Report,* 21 Jan. 2020, https://www.usnews.com/news/best-countries/slideshows/countries-with-the-most-well-developed-public-health-care-system?slide=NaN.
3. Simoes, Pedro. "Who Lives Longest? Top 20 Nations for Life Expectancy." *CBS News,* CBS Interactive, 29 Nov. 2018, https://www.cbsnews.com/pictures/who-lives-longest-cias-top-20-nations-for-life-expectancy/.

Part II

Introduction

1. Anthony, Mitch. "The Terms of Aging." *Financial Advisor Magazine*, Sept. 2017.

Chapter 1

1. DeMasters, Karen. "Health-Care Burden To Top $400,000 For Retirees." *Financial Advisor Magazine*, July 2017.
2. Miller, Mark. "Retirement Spending Triage." *Wealth Management*, June 2019.
3. "Medicare isn't enough for retirees – here's how much extra coverage costs in every state ranked", https://www.businessinsider.com/how-much-medigap-plans-cost-every-state-ranked-2018-6#4-new-jersey-48.
4. Finke, Michael. "Health-Care Costs." *Bottom Line's Guide To A Healthy, Wealthy Retirement*, Bottom Line Inc, 2018, 15.
5. "Medicare Advantage." *Medicare Interactive*, https://www.medicareinteractive.org/get-answers/medicare-basics/medicare-coverage-overview/medicare-advantage.
6. "2019 Employer Health Benefits Survey - Section 1: Cost of Health Insurance." *The Henry J. Kaiser Family Foundation,* 25 Sept. 2019, https://www.kff.org/report-section/ehbs-2019-section-1-cost-of-health-insurance/.

Chapter 2

1. "ADLs and IADLs: Complete Guide To Activities of Daily Living." *Kindly Care*, https://www.kindlycare.com/activities-of-daily-living/.
2. America's Health Insurance Plans Guide to Long-Term Care Insurance, 2004, https://www.in.gov/idoi/files/Guide_to_Long_Term_Care_Insurance.pdf.
3. "Cost of Care Survey 2019." *Genworth,* https://www.genworth.com/aging-and-you/finances/cost-of-care.html.

Chapter 3

1. Franklin, Mary Beth. "Dealing with Widows Requires Empathy and Patience." *Investment News,* 22 July 2019.
2. Protective Life, 2019.
3. "Women Still Part of the Conversation. They Must Be." *Investment News,* 22 July 2019.
4. Faris, Stephanie. "Is a Widow Entitled to a Deceased Husband's Pension Benefits?" *Finance,* 3 May 2019, https://finance.zacks.com/widow-entitled-deceased-husbands-pension-benefits-10751.html.
5. Hersch, Warren S. "Ruark Study: Annuitization Rates Are below 5 Percent." *ThinkAdvisor,* 30 Jan. 2013, https://www.thinkadvisor.com/2013/01/30/ruark-study-annuitization-rates-are-below-5-percen/?slreturn=20190629211033.
6. Max, Sarah. "Don't Let 'Gray Divorce' Derail Your Retirement." *Barron's,* 28 May 2019, https://www.barrons.com/articles/gray-divorce-retirement-51551454226.
7. DePaulo, Bella. "Suddenly Single...How to Start Your New Life." *Bottom Line Personal,* 1 Aug. 2019.

Chapter 4

1. Ehrlich, MD, Amy R. "Caregiver's Checklist." *Bottom Line Personal,* 1 Sept. 2019.
2. "What Is Estate Planning?" *EstatePlanning.com - Powered by WealthCounsel,* https://www.estateplanning.com/What-is-Estate-Planning/.

Chapter 5

1. Slott, CPA, Ed. "Avoid These Costly Mistakes in Retirement Account Withdrawals." *Bottom Line Personal,* 1 Dec. 2018.

Chapter 6

1. Anthony, Mitch. "Harsh Lessons In Modern Con Art." *Financial Advisor Magazine,* Dec. 2017, 37.
2. Ibid., 68.
3. Hurley, Mark P. "Why Client Data Is Gold." *Financial Advisor Magazine,* Dec. 2017.
4. "How Common Is Identity Theft? (Updated 2018) The Latest Stats." *Life-*

Lock Official Site, 2018, https://www.lifelock.com/learn-identity-theft-resources-how-common-is-identity-theft.html.
5. LaPonsie, Maryalene, "10 Things to Do After Your Identity Is Stolen," *U.S. News & World Report,* 8 July 2019, https://money.usnews.com/money/personal-finance/family-finance/articles/things-to-do-after-your-identity-is-stolen.

Chapter 7

1. Dokken, Wade, "Dynamic Withdrawal Rule Simplified," *Financial Advisor Magazine*, Oct. 2015, 37.
2. Nationwide Retirement Institute. *Social Security Outlook,* Nationwide Retirement Institute Conducted by Harris Poll, 2018.
3. Nationwide Retirement Institute. *Social Security Outlook*, Annual Report of the Board of Trustees of the Federal Old-Age and Survivors Insurance and Federal Disability Insurance Trust Funds, 2018.
4. "Educate Clients on the Reality of Social Security Benefits." *Investment News,* 8 July 2019.
5. Nationwide Retirement Institute. *Social Security Outlook,* 2017.
6. Bond, Tyler, "An Ominous Future: A United States Without Pensions," *NPPC,* 3 Jan. 2018, https://protectpensions.org/2018/01/02/united-states-without-pensions/.
7. Pfau, Wade, and Dokken, Wade. "Why 4% Could Fail" *Financial Advisor Magazine,* Sept. 2015, 39.
8. Dokken, Wade, "Dynamic Withdrawal Rule Simplified," *Financial Advisor Magazine*, Oct. 2015, 37.
9. Berger, Robert, "4 Tips for Using Rental Property for Retirement Income" *U.S. News & World Report,* 5 Nov. 2015, https://money.usnews.com/money/blogs/on-retirement/2015/11/05/4-tips-for-using-rental-property-for-retirement-income.
10. Brooks, Rodney, "Never Retire: Why People Are Still Working in Their 70s and 80s," *U.S. News & World Report*, 3 Aug. 2018, https://money.usnews.com/money/retirement/second-careers/articles/never-retire-why-people-are-still-working-in-their-70s-and-80s.

Chapter 9

1. Devine, Colin, and Ken Mungan, "Planning For Retirement Income Within An Increasingly Volatile And Uncertain World," *Alliance for Lifetime Income,* Mar. 2020.

Chapter 10

1. Segal, Troy. "Diversification," *Investopedia,* 6 Mar. 2020, https://www.investopedia.com/terms/d/diversification.asp.
2. Edward Winslow, *Blind Faith, Our Misplaced Trust in the Stock Market, and Smarter, Safer Ways to Invest,* (San Francisco, Berrett-Koehler, 2003) 106-107.
3. Chen, James. "Treasury Inflation-Protected Securities Protect Investors from Inflation." *Investopedia,* 9 Mar. 2020, https://www.investopedia.com/terms/t/tips.asp.

Chapter 11

1. Winslow, *Blind Faith,* 27.
2. Ibid., 43.
3. Ibid., 111.
4. Ibid., 28.
5. "Confirmation Bias." *Wikipedia,* Wikimedia Foundation, 8 Mar. 2020, https://en.wikipedia.org/wiki/Confirmation_bias.
6. Winslow, *Blind Faith,* 35-36.
7. Huang, Nellie S. "Why Your Investment Return May Differ From the Fund Company's Returns." *www.kiplinger.com,* Kiplinger's Personal Finance, 17 May 2019, https://www.kiplinger.com/article/investing/t041-c050-s003-why-your-returns-differ-from-published-fund-return.html.
8. Sommer, Jeff. "Investors Are Usually Wrong. I'm One of Them," *The New York Times,* 26 July 2019, https://www.nytimes.com/2019/07/26/your-money/stock-bond-investing.html.
9. Cussen, Mark P. "How Financial Advice Can Boost Your Returns." *Investopedia,* 25 Jan. 2019, https://www.investopedia.com/articles/personal-finance/102616/how-much-can-advisor-help-your-returns-how-about-3-worth.asp.

Chapter 12

1. "11 Historic Bear Markets." *NBCNews.com,* NBCUniversal News Group, 24 June 2010, http://www.nbcnews.com/id/37740147/ns/business-stocks_and_economy/t/historic-bear-markets/#.Xw-txZ5Kjid.
2. Kenny, Thomas. "Bond Index Returns vs. Stocks and Bonds '80-'18." *Aggregate Bond Index Returns vs. Stocks '80-'18,* The Balance, 17 Nov. 2019, https://www.thebalance.com/stocks-and-bonds-calendar-year-perfor-

mance-417028.
3. Kenny, Thomas. "Historical Performance Data of High-Yield Bonds." *The Balance,* 11 Feb. 2020, https://www.thebalance.com/high-yield-bonds-historical-performance-data-417116.
4. Winslow, Blind Faith, 137.
5. Ibid., 114-115.
6. Ibid., 143.